PRAISE

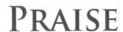

Jill Bausch, a top head-hunter for international organizations, has seen hundreds of women underestimate themselves. *Why Brave Women Win* is the cure to imposter syndrome, showing women how to be themselves and take on the success they deserve. This book should be required reading for all MBA courses worldwide, to help women unleash their power in the workplace.

Professor Peter Piot | Global Health Advisor, former Director, London School of Hygiene and Tropical Medicine, former Executive Director of UNAIDS

This book is inspirational and thought provoking—it's a personal journey with professional advice written in the most honest and open way that just makes you stop and think. I would recommend that all women read this, regardless where they are in their lives or careers.

Tracy Hastain | Business Consultant and 'With Tracy' Podcast Presenter

Jill Bausch's *"Why Brave Women Win"* is not only a joy to read, but it is entertaining! Jill does not talk down to the reader, but confidently leads the reader to success. Listening as a Leader is just one cornerstone of Jill's success, and only one of many tools which will assure success of all its readers. Jill Bausch delivers, with methodical precision, successful and practical solutions dealing with the whole idea of acceptance and the potential within all of us. Jill Bausch's genius is showing the reader that learning from personal experiences, tragedy & joy, only enhances the chances of success in the work-place.

Richard Zieman | Playwright, Author of Pulitzer Prize nominated 'Lighthouses in the Desert'

There are many good books out there which offer sound guidance but no others that I have read in a single sitting. *Why Brave Women Win* is beautifully written, full of practical common sense advice and inspirational material, but it is Jill Bausch's warm encouragement and motivational style that makes this book a must-read.

Pippa Isbell | Founder and Director, Pivotality Leadership & Coaching

This is a must read for any woman, at any stage in their life, as a teenager, student, mother, daughter, manager, leader who wants to learn from the experiences of life to achieve their potential. The book provides hundreds of real-life examples with tools, data and scenarios to allow women to be brave woman and win, whatever their goals. It's a convincing read for a woman to be confident and have openness and ability to learn, therefore as Jill says, to "show-up, stand-up, and speak-up." Jill has a passion to help women and has put pen to paper to help women everywhere.

Dr. Seamus McGardle | Managing Director, SRI Executive Search and Talent Management

Despite the positive changes in our culture, many women feel they don't deserve the success they've earned. Jill Bausch brings decades of experience to bear, with practical advice on how to overcome those false narratives and exercises to help you realize your potential.

Tamara Nall | CEO & Founder, The Leading Niche; *USA Today* and *Wall Street Journal* Bestselling Author of *Business Success Secrets*

Why Brave Women Win is a very rare book—it goes straight to the heart of some of the 21st Century woman's problems and outlines how to solve them. Success isn't instant and, sometimes, it isn't pretty, but the growth you can experience by practicing what Jill Bausch preaches is worth the price!

Shawn Johal | Business Growth Coach, Elevation Leaders, and Bestselling Author of *The Happy Leader*

Can you see yourself in a corporate boardroom? Leading a seminar of top world experts? Overseeing an international aid project? If not, Jill Bausch has some advice for you: If you want to rank among the top professionals, you need to truly believe in yourself. Let *Why Brave Women Win* show you how.

Trissa Tismal-Capili | *USA Today* and *Wall Street Journal* Bestselling Author, and Entrepreneur Flow Expert

When the boss decides, the job goes forward. When the boss understands the strengths and weaknesses of each team member, the team goes forward. Let Jill Bausch's *Why Brave Women Win* teach you how to blend co-worker skill sets in the right proportions and create something brilliant.

Eric Wentz | Bestselling Author of *Zero Two Hundred Hours*

Why Brave Women Win doesn't have all the answers—one book can't have every answer for every woman. Instead, Jill Bausch homes in on the key principles that prevent the success you deserve, and shows you how to chart your own course to your dreams.

Rick Orford | Co-Founder & Executive Producer at Travel Addicts Life, and Bestselling Author of *The Financially Independent Millennial*

Failure is inevitable. Turbulent times are all around us. New levels of preparation will be needed to thrive in this ever-changing world. Jill Bausch has experienced those changes, so let her experience guide you as you learn *Why Brave Women Win*.

Glenn Hopper | CFO, Sandline Discovery, and Bestselling Author of *Deep Finance*

Jill Bausch knows: To-Do list or Not-To-Do list, that is the question. Whether 'tis nobler in the mind to do it all yourself or take arms against a sea of troubles and delegate could mean the difference between just getting the job done and creating something exceptional. *Why Brave Women Win* can show you that difference.

Rick Yvanovich | CEO, TRG

Mohadesa Najumi is quoted as saying "The woman who does not require validation from anyone is the most feared individual on the planet." There is a known plight that hinders people of certain demographics and genders, specifically in relation to what Bausch is seeking to convey in this excellent read. The title is enough to pull you in. Upon delving into *Why Brave Women Win*, you will gain insight as to why the above quote from Najumi is so meaningful here. It takes grit, wisdom, eloquence, and diplomacy to succeed in business let alone in the world. Traits that are often praised in men are shunned for those who were simply born anatomically different. Excellence and bravery are blind to demographics—or at least in reality should be—yet women are often not recognized for the toughness they possess to change nations and business. I thoroughly enjoyed reading the aspects Bausch presented. The touch on empathy in leadership and addressing imposter syndrome to improve leadership are topics that are dear to me and I appreciated Bausch emphasizing their importance as well as highlighting the differences in how men and women deal with them. This is a timely read for both women and men. *Why Brave Women Win* is one book that will live on my bookshelf along with getting passed out to our team members.

Paul Gunn | CEO, KUOG Corporation, and *USA Today* and *Wall Street Journal* Bestselling Author of *Succeed the Right Way*

WHY BRAVE WOMEN WIN

Creating Your Path
to Confidence and Power
in the Workplace

JILL BAUSCH

Leaders
Press

Leaders
Press

ISBN 978-1-63735-152-9 (pbk)
ISBN 978-1-63735-153-6 (ebook)

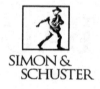

SIMON &
SCHUSTER

Print Book Distributed by Simon & Schuster
1230 Avenue of the Americas
New York, NY 10020

Library of Congress Control Number: 2021924651

DEDICATION

To Josephine, Hannah, Pippa, and Flo, the bravest women I have had the joy to know and who are an inspiration to me every day. And to Harrison, who bravely reminds me there is always hope in adversity. Without all of them and their endless support, this book would not be written.

CONTENTS

PREFACE

Women can sometimes get so lost in what is expected of them, they try to do everything. Everything for themselves and for everyone around them. Some women equate action and "help" to their own self-esteem and how much others will love them. But, sometimes, they do so much that they make others dependent and themselves co-dependent. Does this resonate with you?

If it does, ask yourself, "What am I doing now to create what I **do** want and avoid what I **don't** want?"

I think of women's minds like a row of ping pong balls. Each little ball has a part of her life emblazoned on it: children by name, best friends by name, work, pets, partner, hair and body upkeep, money, tasks, feeding the family, and a zillion other elements of everyone's lives. We're always scooting the little balls forward in our minds and, when one is left behind, we make a special effort to scoot that up to the current baseline by caretaking that element.

On the other hand, I think many men's minds are like a football emblazoned with WORK in giant letters, sitting in the middle of a field with lots of marbles on the sidelines. The marbles are wife/partner, children, sports, sex, food, and other things. But, if the big WORK ball does not move forward, the marbles don't shift either. Often, the football is the only one that shifts.

Women don't think or behave this way. For many men, if their work disappears, their whole identity is shattered—what he does is who he thinks he is. When a women's work disappears, she finds a replacement, but her safety net is still usually there. She has all the other balls of a similar magnitude and size and importance. This is why science shows that men die earlier in almost every society around the globe. This is why they suffer more from divorce. This is why, in most cultures, when a separation threatens us, it is overwhelmingly the woman who makes the final choice to separate or divorce.

In so many cases, women just leave (often silently) or stay physically, but quit trying. Exasperated with trying to get their male partner to understand what they feel, women sometimes cannot penetrate the massive football exterior that is some men's self-image. Without it, they don't know who they are.

What will make men's priorities more balanced? What will make them more emotionally intelligent, more caring, softer, more vulnerable? Is it nature or nurture? Is it how we raise them? Did I teach my son the same way I taught my daughter? Can we teach ourselves to be brave? Can we teach our children to be brave if it does not come naturally? I believe we can because I know *Why Brave Women Win*.

CHAPTER 1
SHE WHO DARES, WINS

INTRODUCTION — THE LOW IN THE HIGH LIFE

JUNE 1994

I am sitting in the hot tub on the roof of the Meurice Hotel in Paris, in the presidential suite, alone.

In the last hour, the expert staff at this 5-star+ hotel have delivered a two-foot ice sculpture, a bottle of Tattinger Champagne and a tray of foie-gras to my suite. I'm Director of Marketing Communications for Intercontinental Hotels for Europe, Middle East, and Africa. When I stay in one of the hotels, they bestow their best treats on me because it bodes well for them if I "experience" the exemplary attention they bestow on guests. But every time some gloved butler brings something else, with each rap on the door, I feel emptier.

In every hotel, in all these exotic locations around the globe, it's the same. In all these places, the 5-star excess is giving me a 1-star feeling in my gut. The contradictions in the world are troubling me because the poor get poorer, the rich get richer, and the divide gets wider every year. I know I'm lucky to have the job, live the life, and all that comes with it, plus a supportive husband

and two small children at home but, suddenly, it's not enough. The job is increasingly meaningless to me. I don't want my legacy to be a solitary life feathering my nest without purpose. I've been feeling this way for a while and I know something must change. I've spent 10 years in senior roles in Hyatt, Marriott and Intercontinental Hotels and been all around the world. Increasingly, that just isn't enough.

But how do I change it? Do I just walk away? And to what?

JANUARY 1995

I'm sitting in the Rueben's Hotel in London, attending a hotel marketing conference. I've reached the point where the reason for marketing luxury hotels completely eludes me, and I go home every night feeling like life is passing but I'm not learning, not growing. I've hit my limit at this conference, so I leave the conference room, head to the lobby of the hotel and order an expensive coffee while sitting by the hotel's front windows, which face Buckingham Palace.

Absentmindedly, I pick up a London magazine I would never normally read and flip to the ads in the back. There, I find an advertisement for a job in the Department for International Development (DFID), the agency of the British government that bestows monetary aid on developing countries in need. They are looking for marketing experts to train in social marketing. I've never heard of social marketing but quickly learn that it's marketing products and services for social good—with an emphasis on halting the growing HIV/AIDS epidemic which is ravaging Africa and Asia—by creating marketing and education programs for poor people at risk of contracting AIDS.

A little quick research scares me: Hundreds of thousands of children in Asia and Africa were already AIDS orphans. About 1.2 million people die from AIDS every year across Africa—out of 1.7 million worldwide. Although antiretroviral drug treatments can seriously decrease HIV-related deaths, drug supplies in Africa are woefully insufficient. In some years, half the AIDS population gets no treatment.

I am instantly energized by the idea of this new job; one I know I can do with my whole heart and soul. The ad says the government will train those they accept in the areas of sexual health, social marketing, and working within aid agencies, then employ them in British government aid programs.

Then came the bad news, I found some roadblocks. Candidates must have the following:

1. British Citizenship. (I did not, although I was married to a British citizen.)
2. Commercial FMCG experience. (Another hurdle—FMCG stands for "fast-moving consumer goods" and hotels certainly are not.)
3. Professional experience in women's health issues. (Besides actually being a woman, I had none.)
4. Experience in poverty-stricken countries in Africa and Asia. (The closest I could get was a visit with my sister to Nepal a few years prior, when she adopted my niece. My title might be Director of

Marketing Communications Public Relations for Europe, Middle East, and Africa, but our hotels are in major cities—Cairo, Amman, Delhi—where the poor congregate outside the doors to beg. Hardly the experience they were seeking.)

Still, I tore the ad out, downed my coffee, and, instead of returning to my office, I went home and applied for the job. I later found out they had six places to fill and over 600 applicants. My chances were definitely not looking good.

On the London tube (the British name for the subway) heading home, I thought, *I don't have anything they have asked for, but I do have two things they didn't ask for.*

1. Confidence.
2. The ability to learn anything that I put my mind to, if I care enough about it.

So, I waited. And waited. And, one evening, I came home from work to hear a phone message thanking me for the application, but sorry, DFID said I did not meet any of the criteria they were seeking. I listened to the message, and as I heard it, I simply sat down and cried. My four-year-old daughter, Hannah, was next to me when I heard the message. I excused myself from her to go to my bedroom and have a real wail.

A few minutes later, mid-sob, there was a gentle *tap-tap-tap* at my bedroom door. Hannah came in wearing her fuzzy pajamas, holding a bowl into which she'd tipped a whole bottle of green olives, one of my favorite foods.

She said, "Mummy, I know you're sad and I don't know why, but I hope this makes you feel better."

I stewed in my sadness overnight and tried to reconcile this lost opportunity. Then I decided to use the power I had. I pulled out my two secret weapons: confidence and my ability to learn.

I rang DFID the next morning and asked who oversaw this program. To my surprise, they gave me a name. Even more remarkably, when I asked to speak to him, they put me through.

A kindly male voice asked if he could help me and, when I asked if I could speak to the head of hiring for this post, he replied, "That's me."

I thanked him for taking my call, told him my application had been turned down but that I felt I had a lot to offer. Knowing that a personal meeting face to face is almost always best, I asked him if he would give me 15 minutes to talk if I came to his office, with the promise that I would not stay longer, I would not stalk or pester or plead with him when he said the meeting was over.

Astonishingly, he agreed.

I planned those 15 minutes very carefully and, on the appointed day, sat down with the gentleman. The details of the conversation are unimportant, except that, when I was done, he started a conversation that lasted, all-in-all, about two hours. I left his office with the job in hand. Life then pivoted for me enormously. I was now moving in the right direction. Over the next two years that I worked for DFID, and the following 10 years as CEO of Futures Group Europe, I had tremendous opportunities to learn, to grow, to give, and to take back some of my own power—power I felt I'd lost in the grind of my hotel PR life, which had lost its meaning for me.

THE BASICS

Before you get anywhere near a job interview, before you do anything, set yourself up for success. In the Meurice Hotel in Paris, I asked myself three questions: "How do I change it? Do I just walk away? And to what?"

That first question is the reason for this book and we'll explore answers to that question in the chapters to come.

The answer to the second question is, "No!" Unless you're in a toxic or dangerous situation, and, if that's the case, the answer is still no—you **run**, fast and far! Do not allow an employment situation to risk your health or safety—no paycheck is worth it. I mention this because that's where I was heading. I said to myself, "I don't want my legacy to be a solitary life, feathering my nest without purpose." One of the hallmarks of the Millennial generation is their quest for purpose, for meaningful employment. I didn't know that at the time, but they were on to something I was unconsciously beginning to figure out.

That last question is the key and is the other side of the coin of question two. Sometimes, people get so fed up that they just quit. That is not always the best plan. Don't run away **from everything**, run **to something, even if it is an idea that you haven't realized yet**. I considered leaving the hotel world before I had a place to go, but I didn't go until I was inspired by another direction.

What will be your new direction?

Answering that will mean some self-analysis, research, time, etc. Do it! A wise man once said, "If you don't know where you're going, you'll probably end up somewhere else." What are the odds that it'll be the place you want to be in?

As you're doing the job search and, definitely, when you're prepping for an interview:

1. Be polite but be persistent. Understand the difference between **confidence** and **arrogance**; the difference between **persistent** and **pushy**.
2. Don't just see what you **don't** have, see what you **do** have.
3. **Packaging** is fine, **BS-ing** and **lying** are not. Don't say you know it if you don't, but say you'll learn it and that you're great at learning. Have some examples ready to share of how you've learned and become effective. And then get great at what they need and do it well.
4. People **want** to fill the job. It's their **job** to fill the job. But they also **need** to fill the job with the best qualified candidate. That's also part of their job. Make it **easy** for them to feel they are in trusted hands if they hire you.

5. If you don't feel confident, **find a mentor and mirror her**. Imagine a role model, someone you admire, role play in your head how they would handle it. How would they hold themselves, look, and speak? What would they wear? Mirror them. I'm often asked if it's possible to teach confidence. Yes, if you mirror it enough, it becomes a habit. While this habit develops, you may fear being exposed as a fraud. If you do, you may have what is called "imposter syndrome." It's a common problem and we'll address it in a later chapter, but for now, rest assured that it will dissipate. You can, and will, with the right mentoring and practice, become what you can only now pretend to be.

"Imposter syndrome"—perhaps just a fancy term for a lack of self-confidence—is an old story among women. (Men are not immune to it, but men and women deal with it in different ways, and it affects substantially more females than males.) Christine Lagarde, president of the European Central Bank, and former head of the International Monetary Fund (IMF), said, in a *Forbes* interview[1]:

> "There's plenty of that still going around and it's very, very unfortunate and very sad. ... [N]ot only is it offensive to those who have to

---

[1] Joan Michelson, "Christine Lagarde on Sexism, Climate Change and the Future of Work, Post-Covid," *Forbes.com*, Jersey City, NJ: Forbes Media LLC, 2021. https://www.forbes.com/sites/joanmichelson2/2021/04/30/christine-lagarde-on-sexism-climate-change-and-the-future-of-work-post-covid/?sh=130008f4265d, accessed 6 May 2022.

bear the brunt of it and put up with that, but it's a huge waste of opportunity and it's a huge waste of talent. ... I mean, it does take the form of the 'sofa-gate' kind of business. ... But it also takes the form of those sort of lack of access, discrimination, hinted biases, dismissive comments, and it goes on and on. ... from an economy point of view, only looking at it from that angle, it's a huge waste of talent."

So, when you sit in a board room with 20 or 25 people and only one or two are female, it's natural to wonder, "Are we supposed to be here?"

Centuries of wrong thinking say "No!" Some still say it, and they say it forcefully. The real answer is "Yes." How do I know that? Because you're there. People don't just walk into corporate or government leadership. You apply or run, and you or your campaign are vetted. You must convince a group of selectors—managers, stockholders, or voters—that you're the right person for that job.

When they say, "Yes," **believe them**!

CHAPTER 2
WHY TOUGH EMPATHY MATTERS

*"Between two evils, I always pick the one
I never tried before."*

—Mae West

INTRODUCTION — THE STOCKBRIDGE SYNDROME

When I was 15, my mother told me (again!) that I was disruptive to the family—a bad influence on my four brothers and sisters. She was right.

At 15, I was doing everything I shouldn't do—smoking heaps of pot, skipping school or attending classes stoned. I consistently ignored everything my parents had to say about what I could do, where I could go, and who I could see. Mom told me I was being sent to a boarding school because she couldn't cope with me at home.

She had clearly taken her cue from school counselors and shrinks, who advised her to remove me to keep the rest of the family sane. She showed me information from three schools and told me I had to choose one. The following week, she insisted we drive to see all three schools. We left our little town in upstate New York and crossed into Massachusetts. After more than four hours of driving, we arrived. Two campuses reminded me of military academies, which scared and repulsed me—after, all, I was way too cool for that kind of school! The third was Stockbridge School. At first glance, the place looked like an upscale hippie commune. All the students had long hair and wore ripped jeans. The stench of pot pervaded every moment of the campus tour. Forced to choose one of the three, I naturally chose Stockbridge.

Looking back, I think Mom gave me no alternative but to choose that school and, in the end, it got me unstuck. Did she know I would choose Stockbridge? Parents are usually a lot smarter than their teenagers give them credit for. Among the choices I was given, of course I would've chosen Stockbridge. It was a no-brainer.

A few weeks later, Mom drove me back to Stockbridge and dropped me off for the start of winter term. I could see the relief in her eyes. I was assigned a room and roommate, then my mother said a swift goodbye and abruptly started her four-hour journey home.

My roommate, I learned quickly, was typical of the "students" at this wild and expensive place. She was a trust-fund baby, sent there so her parents could be rid of her until she grew up. Within 20 minutes of Mom's departure, roomie pulled out a joint and asked if I wanted to share. (As the weeks passed, I saw her light many more, including one every morning, before she even got out of bed. She awoke, reached for her fix, lighted it, and smoked the whole thing.)

Roomie and I had a lot in common. First and foremost, we were both incorrigible. But between us there was an important difference. I had loving parents—they cared about me, but couldn't cope with me. As we got acquainted, I learned that all my roommate's parents had to do was pay the bills, and that was all they did. I also learned that many of our classmates were in the same boat as roomie. Their parents weren't just absent physically, they were **all-but-nonexistent** in their children's lives.

And it showed, even on that first day: As roomie and I shared that first joint, trading stories of how rotten our families were for sending us here, in walked another 15-year-old girl who had a boyfriend in prison near Boston. (We actually hitchhiked to Beantown to see him some weeks later!) Others joined the impromptu dorm room get-together, including a guy who admitted to me he's gay and came here looking for sex. He found it. Since arriving in September, he'd had lots of sex, with both students and teachers.

Suddenly, about an hour into our drug-induced groove, roomie pulls off her tee shirt—no bra—and clearly loves the attention her nudity was attracting.

At that point, a tiny light went on in the back of my head, so dimly that I barely noticed it, but it was there. At 15, I was a juvenile delinquent but not a complete imbecile. I had stopped short of promiscuity, hard drugs, and acts of total stupidity, although my parents would disagree on that last point. Well, over the next several weeks, I saw so much crass, vulgar and just plain frightening behaviour—from both teachers and students—that I actually got scared. Is this my destiny, I asked myself—no path, no achievement, no family, no home?

No thanks!

I decided to hitchhike the 300 miles home to upstate New York. I'd begun to value that home, to miss my family, to question my behaviour, and to promise myself that I would straighten up if I was allowed to stay. Sometimes, when the gift is taken away, you value the gift more.

When I finally arrived home and walked in the front door, Mom did not throw her arms around me in an act of love. She simply looked up and said, "What are you doing here and how did you get here?" When I tried to explain that I was done with that place and wanted to come back, to be a real part of the family, she simply said, "No." She called Greyhound Bus Lines to find out when the next bus would leave for Stockbridge and put me into the car to drive me to the station.

I had just enough time to grab some clothes from my old bedroom and steal a bottle of Canadian Club bourbon (my mother's favourite tipple) from my parents' liquor cabinet. With the bourbon secreted on the bottom of a paper grocery bag and covered with my clothes, I was again thrown out of my home. Cool and aloof, Mom put me on the bus back to school. I was angry and hurt—only much later would I understand that my mother was as angry and as hurt as I could ever be, because of the trauma I'd caused her. I crashed myself down onto the bus seat and dropped the bag on the floor. The bourbon bottle broke, soaking my clothes, and filling the bus with the stench of alcohol. My fellow passengers were not pleased.

Throughout the rest of the term, my mother implored me, via handwritten letters, not to attempt this again. They loved me, she assured, but they insisted that I finish my sophomore high school year at Stockbridge.

When the school year ended, they allowed me to return home. Our high school created a plan that made it possible for me to complete my junior and senior years together. (I think they just wanted me to go away.) During that year, I got straight As, did not drink a drop of booze, lost 25 pounds and graduated.

That was possible because my life had changed in one vital way—I became terrified of the consequences of my previous bad choices. But I don't believe events would've worked out as well as they did if my parents had let me stay when I hitchhiked home. The light had come on inside me, but it hadn't burned bright enough or long enough for me to fully see the end of the road I'd put myself on. It took the full term for the lesson to burn itself deep enough into my psyche to affect me permanently.

I had, for the first time, experienced tough empathy.

Sympathy vs. Empathy

Sympathy, noun

"The act or state of feeling sorrow or compassion for another: [as in] *I can do no more than express my deep sympathy for you in your loss.*"[2]

Empathy, noun.

"The psychological identification with or vicarious experiencing of the emotions, thoughts, or attitudes of another: [as in] *She put an arm around her friend's shoulders and stood by her in silent empathy.*"[3]

Sympathy is feeling sorrow for someone, "Too bad you're going through that"—but to remain emotionally aloof from their situation.

Empathy is thinking, "How must it feel to go through that?"—to try and put yourself in that other person's shoes, to understand their situation from their perspective.

Tough Empathy

In the context of a professional environment, tough empathy balances the business needs of the organization with the personal needs of the employees.

Every business must have goals, procedures, policies, and so on. Quality organizations recognize that their people are vital to meeting those goals, and allow

---

[2] "Sympathy," *Dictionary.com*, accessed 2 June 2022.
[3] "Empathy," *Dictionary.com*, accessed 2 June 2022.

some flexibility in the procedures, policies, and so on, so that the people perform at their peak efficiency and profitability.

(I know, that sounds so obvious, you might wonder why it even needs to be stated. Sadly, many organizations get so focused on profit that they lose sight of everything else and become hostile or toxic workspaces. Even in the 21st Century, too many organizations have this attitude. You should really try to avoid working for them.)

We've all heard stories of supervisors or managers who are absolute taskmasters: "I don't care about your personal problems; I'm only interested in results!" is a cliché movie line that establishes a character as a taskmaster. Some of these people almost qualify as sociopaths. They're not killers, they simply become so focused on the end result, the bottom line, the perks, the money, the profit, whatever ... that they lose their humanity, at least as far as the well-being of co-workers is concerned.

On the flip side, some supervisors or managers are absolute pushovers. They're so empathetic, they listen to everybody's problems, and say, "Sure, take another day off. All well and good."

That only works until we suddenly find that the job won't get done on time or on budget, or it doesn't meet specifications, goals aren't met and the business is failing.

"Tough empathy" is the sweet spot between the two. A supervisor or manager who gets this concept might say, "My team is like family, I care about what happens to you. I know you have lives outside the office and I respect those other obligations. However, we still have to deliver on our goals." That supervisor will build a safety net into their organizational procedures and policies so that, if one employee "fails" (through their own fault or due to circumstances outside their control), the rest of the team can step in, fill the gap and get the job done while helping that teammate deal with their situation.

In its simplest form, it's about balance and creating a cohesive, mutually-supportive business team.

FINDING BALANCE

How does a person find that balance, personally or in business? It requires a lot of introspection. You can start by setting aside some time and asking yourself some questions:

- What do you **need** to achieve?
- What do you **want** to achieve?
- What **don't you need** to achieve?
- When do you **have to achieve** these things or not?

Those are specific, and to some, a little confusing. You'll probably need to do more than think about the answers. You'll need to ponder the answers to really understand your personal priorities. For example, many GenXers and Millennials are more interested in the contribution they can make to the world than in the paycheck they get for it. They'll accept a mid-range salary in a company with an agenda that matches theirs, instead of a hefty salary in a company with no agenda beyond providing a product or service to their clientele.

Obviously, in the arena of job hunting, this would require serious research by you, the job applicant, on the companies you may want to join. You'd need to enter an interview with questions that'll tell you about the supervisors or managers you'll work with and the company's social, political, environmental, or other goals.

In my current role as Director of Search and Leadership for SRI Executive, we understand tough empathy and practice it. It is part of the ethos of the organisation. SRI Executive was started more than 20 years ago by Helen McGardle in Dublin. A short time later, her husband Seamus joined her in the business and together they have built SRI into one of the world's leading Executive Search and Talent Management agencies serving international development and philanthropic organisations. We source and pre-qualify potential senior executives, mostly for international organisations. Our clients expect the best quality people, but sometimes we have to practice tough empathy. I might have to tell them, for example, "We need to give this person space and time. They recently suffered a family tragedy, so they weren't at their best during that interview." Clients generally understand and will accommodate. (That is another aspect of practicing tough empathy.)

We recognize that these high-caliber candidates are whole people and we do psychometric leadership assessments on almost everybody. These assessments are very valuable because they're cost effective and highly accurate as to how a person will deal with their team, expressing themselves, being inclusive, and many other essential elements in good leadership.

Emotional Intelligence relates directly to tough empathy. We now have excellent psychometric tools, available in many forms, which are robustly researched and produce very accurate results. I'm certified in several of these tools and I use them all the time. It helps also that I'm a certified executive coach. I interpret these psychometrics and they can give you, the supervisor or manager, an assessment of where you are in your path to becoming an inspiring and adept leader. That becomes a great baseline for your leadership development plan, if you're introspective enough and sufficiently motivated to improve. If you're open enough and brave enough, you can say, "Okay, I'm going to have my own assessment done." You'll find there will be elements where you will be able to say, "Look I'm great at these elements of leadership and communications, but I have some work to do here or there."

Some people are more naturally inclined to be empathetic or to correctly use tough empathy than others. By knowing your current skill level, you have a baseline for what additional training you need and skill sets you need to develop to reach that sweet spot in your organization.

EI/EQ

Businesses in the postwar generations, my parents' generation, were often run by former military officers and, often, with an equally demanding leadership style. Today, corporate leadership needs a different methodology. There are still a few executives who think in those militaristic or authoritarian terms, but these attitudes are counterproductive and rapidly disappearing. In their place, modern executives are expected to show increased "emotional intelligence," also called "emotional quotient," in addition to their technical skills.

Emotional intelligence (EI) and Emotional Quotient (EQ) aren't difficult concepts, in theory, but the practice can be challenging. Simply put, anyone with a solid EI/EQ understands their own emotions and how to deal with them in the business world. Ask yourself:

- Do you understand how you're affected by what happens around you?
- Do you understand how your reactions may affect other people?

Some people are often confused about the EI/EQ concept. It isn't, "Are you emotional?" or "Do you publicly display your emotions?"

In looking at EI/EQ, a leader might say, "Well, I have a big staff, and I have to be the boss. And I don't want to divulge too much about myself, emotionally." This is absolutely appropriate; a certain level of professional boundary is necessary to establish and maintain the respect of peers and juniors. But that comment shows that person has yet to learn about what emotional intelligence really is.

In larger terms, EI/EQ is the ability to understand, use, and manage your own emotions in positive ways to relieve stress, communicate effectively, empathize with others, overcome challenges and defuse conflict. Emotional Intelligence helps you build stronger relationships, succeed at school and work, and achieve your career and personal goals. It can also help you to connect with your feelings, turn intention into action, and make informed decisions about what matters most to you.[4]

EI/EQ doesn't mean giving too much of yourself. It is the awareness of how you react to others and how you see co-workers as feeling and thinking people. Effective leaders allow themselves to be emotional privately. They process it, then come back and give the public their best selves, communicating constructively and listening more than talking. There's a lot of research showing that people who are successful in a holistic way—not just at making a lot of money—have high emotional intelligence. In fact, research shows that your EI/EQ level is a much better indicator of professional success than your Intelligence Quotient (IQ), long

---

[4] Dr. Jeanne Segal, Melinda Smith, Lawrence Robinson & Jennifer Shubin, "Improving Emotional Intelligence (EQ)," *HelpGuide.org*. Santa Monica, CA: HelpGuideOrg Int'l, 2021, accessed 2 June 2022.
https://www.helpguide.org/articles/mental-health/emotional-intelligence-eq.htm#:~:text=What%20is%20emotional%20intelligence%20or,overcome%20challenges%20and%20defuse%20conflict, accessed 2 June 2022.

thought to be the benchmark of your brain's power and capacity. Businesses are coming to understand that EI/EQ can change, often with minimal effort, for those interested in self-improvement that leads to professional success.

As Bob Marley famously said, "Some people are so poor, all they have is money."

EXAMPLES

THE AU PAIR

I've always worked. I took a couple of months off when each of my children were born, but then I went back to the job. To make that work, like so many people here in England, I always had an *au pair*, many of them French, most of them on a one-year contract, hoping to improve their English with a family in Great Britain.

So, this one fine day in June, a young woman of about 22 arrived from France to be our new *au pair*. She was taking a break from university and wanted to learn English before she went on to do whatever she was going to do in life. She arrived on a weekend and we agreed with her that she'd begin work on Monday morning, after getting used to the household. Sunday evening, we reviewed the plan: "You get up, you dress the kids, I'll be around to help you." We went through the whole family routine and her responsibilities.

When I got up the next morning, there was no sign of her. We then lived in a tall Victorian house with a bedroom and a bathroom on the top floor where the *au pairs* lived. The middle floor had family bedrooms. The public spaces were the ground floor. I didn't hear her, there was no sign of her. I finally went upstairs as my husband headed out to work. I needed to get on my way to work as well.

So, I went upstairs and knocked on her door. She was in there; I could hear her sobbing her heart out through the closed door.

"Are you okay?" I said through the closed door.

Her English was limited, but it was good enough. "I'm homesick."

"I'm sorry you're homesick, it must be really hard for you." I paused. "But I have to go to work. So, are you going to be able to do what we discussed yesterday?"

"I can't. I can't. I can't cope. I can't cope," she said between sobs.

"Okay, well, I'll dress the kids. I'll call in late for work. I'll take the kids to daycare. But you have today to decide whether you can cope or not. If you can't, I understand, but then you're going to have to go back to France tomorrow, because I have a family to run. If you can cope then you're welcome to stay, but I can only give you today."

She sobbed some more and said, "Okay, okay."

About five o'clock that evening, after picking up the kids, we came home. The *au pair* had cleaned up, dinner was going, she was ready to roll. She'd made up her mind, and was one of the best *au pairs* we ever had. During the months that followed, we talked about her very rocky start and she had a few more rough days in her time with us, but she made it.

That first morning, I felt I had to be tough. I had a household, a family, and a business to manage, but I also had to care about her. She was a human being in pain. I could've shouted, "Get up and get to work!" but that would've been the end of it. She couldn't do it that Monday morning. So, I said, in effect, 'I'm sorry. You get a day, but only one day because that's what the job requires.' As it turned out, she didn't even need the whole day—she was on the job that afternoon. She stayed the year plus six months and was a great *au pair* and a lovely person. I was really sorry to see her go.

THE BOARD MEMBER

In an earlier part of my career, I was Chief Executive Officer of Futures Group Europe. My direct boss was the corporation's chairman of the board. A gentleman who served as a member of the global board was in the HQ office in Bath, England one day. He was in in his late 40s, some years older than myself and, as a board member, technically my superior at that time.

As we discussed some business issues, I was somewhat offended over the way he expressed something to me. Thus far, he and I had gotten along pretty well, but he noticed the tone of the conversation change.

"What's up with this conversation?" he asked

"Well, you kind of hurt my feelings," I said.

"You know, I care about your feelings, but you need to have thicker skin. You need to separate hurt feelings from business objectives."

This was a wake-up call for me. As I thought it over, I realized he was right—this is work. I needed to be more aware. We all need to be aware enough to ask, "Did he/she intend to hurt my feelings or is this just him/her making the work happen?" Then, we need skin thick enough to forgive, to forget, and to move on.

That was a very valuable day. He used tough empathy to teach me, "I care about you. But this isn't about your feelings. This is about us getting the job done." I later served on that board with him as peers, and we worked very well together.

PRACTICAL FACTORS

How do supervisors and managers demonstrate EI/EQ and tough empathy? A few suggestions:

KEY PERFORMANCE INDICATORS

Most businesses have Key Performance Indicators (KPIs). I've always used these as a metaphorical contract. My team members and I agree to KPIs for each of them, so we both know what should happen.

Each team member takes the lead for their individual KPIs. If they need my help, I have an open door, but I expect them to deliver, unless they give me reasons in advance why they can't. If it's due on Monday, don't come to me on Monday saying, "I didn't get it done." Tell me on Friday or Thursday or even Wednesday, "I am not going to make Monday and this is why." I can work with that. I remind my team that we have to deliver on the goals, but I try to give them reasonable expectations.

DON'T PULL RANK

I don't use a hierarchical approach to management. That is, I don't pull rank or assume all the power.

I might say, "We have a conference call with these officials from these international organizations to discuss a problem that involves those organizations. So, I think it might be a good idea for me to lead the discussion."

I could just as easily say, "I know better than you because you're junior to me." Or, less harshly, "I'll always take the lead in discussions because I'm the manager." Lots of people think this is the way to go, and, sometimes, it needs to be. However, there's an old proverb, "The best way to get a promotion is to train your successor." I agree—all supervisors have an obligation to train their people to take over for them, and that includes letting them take charge for a day or a project.

You may have heard the old military proverb, "No battle plan ever survives the first contact with the enemy." In the larger sense, few plans ever survive first contact with reality. You have to have backups, alternatives, options to turn to when things don't happen exactly the way you thought they would.

PULL RANK

I'm not afraid to pull rank, but only when I have to. I'm paid to be in charge. I'm paid to make decisions and take responsibility for those decisions, so I expect my team to back me up.

While we were screening prospects to run a United Nations organization, my number two on this project was very good, but still learning the ropes. One day, we were in a video conference with representatives from several member states of the organization. I put forward some information about a certain candidate and she disagreed with me—on the call with the member state reps! This is not the way we work. We don't have the senior say, "Here's my assessment of this person," only to have the junior say during the call, "I don't really think that."

This wasn't about my ego getting bruised. My ego was fine. It was about conducting business on a professional level and presenting a cohesive report to the client. Disagreements within our team decrease our credibility to our clients. That's a fast track to not getting return business.

So, in a situation like this, two things need to happen: First, you need to have your co-workers' back. I didn't embarrass her publicly. I left that agenda item and moved quickly to the next. Second, after the call, I connected with her immediately. We got together on a video call and I said, "You're learning and I want you to learn, but there are people that have more time in this role, more stripes. In this case, that's me. My job is to lead the project and provide a united front so the clients have confidence that they're going to hire the right candidate. They don't want to hear me say one thing, immediately followed by you saying the opposite. And I can't allow that because it jeopardizes our client relationship. When we're vetting candidates, you can present any disagreement to me and I will listen to you privately. When the decision is made, though, you need to back my decision." It was tough empathy at work.

CONCLUSION

It would be easy to say, "Tough empathy means giving people what they need, not what they want," but I don't think that's precisely accurate.

Tough empathy has been practiced on me, and I've practiced it on others. After the fact, after I've had time to digest the lesson and integrate it, I find myself saying, "That made me a better person."

When that board member said to me, "You need to have thicker skin; you need to separate hurt feelings from business objectives," it made me a better executive and leader. So, I don't think tough empathy is simply what they need. I believe that, eventually, the recipient needs to think, "Yeah, okay. I needed that; I just didn't know I needed it. But I'm lucky I got it."

Elvis Presley's last girlfriend before he died was asked what she thought killed him. She said, "Elvis didn't hear enough 'No's.'" Everyone said yes to Elvis all the time. He got what he wanted when he wanted it and look what it ultimately cost him.

CHAPTER 3

FROM IMPOSTER SYNDROME TO AUTHENTICITY

Like a small boat on the ocean
Sending big waves into motion
Like how a single word can make a heart open
I might only have one match, but I can make an
explosion

And all those things I didn't say,
Wrecking balls inside my brain
I will scream them loud tonight,
Can you hear my voice this time?

This is my fight song
Take back my life song
Prove I'm alright song
My power's turned on

Starting right now I'll be strong
I'll play my fight song
And I don't really care if nobody else believes
'Cause I've still got a lot of fight left in me.

　　　　　　　　　—Rachel Platton, "Fight Song"

Introduction — Posting the Banns

The little hovercraft holds about 30 people and sits deflated on the beach like a spent jellyfish, facing the Isle of Wight, a nautical mile away. A crusty old chap in a faded blue uniform takes my ticket, allowing me to trudge over the sand and up a rickety portable stairway onto the craft. Once all passengers are safely on, children, their parents, and I scurry for the window seats, the stairs are kicked away as the engines roar up, a head-ringing noise starts and the hovercraft blows up from the bottom, teetering back and forth until it is fully inflated, and the air influx stabilizes it (sort of) from side to side. As it backs itself into the water of the Solent (a narrow strait off the English Channel) humming loudly, it spins round, gathers momentum, and travels a few feet above the water's surface by the force of the air against the sea. The ride you're in for is entirely dependent on the state of the sea, because it mirrors the waves below you. If it's rough, hang on, because the bouncing and weaving can be like a roller coaster ride.

When the big rubber ring under your bum hits each wave, you fly upwards, only constrained by a seatbelt. The wave then crashes with a boom against the windows. Repeat 100 times and you have crossed the Solent, landing on the Isle of Wight with a sore midriff in tow. You'll spill out of the craft onto the sand on the other side. The Solent is known not only as one of the busiest bodies of water in the world, but also one of the roughest. If you love roller coasters, take the Hovercraft from Southsea to Ryde in January. It's cheaper, safer, wilder, and more fun than any carnival ride.

On that clear, blue-sky June morning, the weekend after my move from the USA to England, I set off for the Isle of Wight ("The Island," to the locals) with the man I am to marry, Peter. It was something we would do most every weekend during our ten-year marriage.

Leaving our flat in London, we'd pack the car and drive south through the green stockbroker belt of lushly wooded Surrey and the tiny post-card villages of the Meon Valley, Hampshire, stop for morning coffee or a late afternoon glass of wine if we took off on Friday evening. There were a thousand picturesque, thatched-roof pubs in English hamlets along the route to the south coast. Massive hanging baskets spilling with flowers swayed invitingly in front of the pubs as we meandered along the valleys bursting with colour.

In summer throughout the English countryside, rapeseed fields grow ever more golden, and we would come over the crest of the hill to be greeted by a mustard-gold blanket shimmering in fields in front of us. I loved these drives and so did my soon-to-be husband. Once we reached the tiny seaside port of Southsea, we'd sling our bags onto the hovercraft and set off to that charming anachronistic isle. When Peter's parents died some years earlier, Peter and his only brother inherited a Georgian Manor House perched on a hill, with spectacular views of the sea, long green lawns, and a short walk down the hill, to his beloved 'home' village.

Our destination was Seaview, a village perched on the sea front, with boats littering the tiny front lawns of cottages facing the single lane that runs in and out of the village. In summer, the village is inhabited largely by wealthy upper-class English who have second houses there and have been coming there for generations. Some of the more senior of those now live full time in the village, retired from professional careers in London—executives from banking, government, or industry. But whatever they did for a living, they were not used to, and were often clearly uncomfortable with, having an outsider in their closed community. Seaview is like American summer camp for kids. If you know people, the welcome is endless. If not, it can be hard work. Years later, when I was known there, if a new person was brought into the social set in Seaview, I immediately took them under my wing them to help them feel at home because I never forgot how difficult it was for me.

When we're brought up in America—"the melting pot"—most of us are taught to accept others unless given reason not to. Diversity of nationalities, religions, and cultures are part of our history. Although England is also remarkably diverse, acceptance of others is not so natural to their culture, quite the opposite, in fact, for many English. One must allow time to be accepted and you must earn that acceptance. Until then, you are inevitably and relentlessly examined until you prove worthy. Of course, I did not know that back then.

When the English first meet you (and Americans are usually unaware of this), they immediately position you in the social pecking order according to your accent. The English accent (actually hundreds of regional and local speech patterns) contains a plethora of information to be gleaned about you as soon as you say a word.

Your accent and mode of speech will inform the English listener wordlessly all about you: Working class? Middle Class? Upper class? Northern? Yorkshire? Cornwall? The answer lies in your speech, enabling the listener to make many assumptions about you, your background, wealth, status and education ... in short, where are you in the pecking order? Are you the same class as they?

Even with devoted and sustained elocution lessons, it is almost impossible to transcend this way of establishing credentials. After living in England for 18 years, I became adept at pegging accents and giving a very accurate account of a person's background after only a few sentences. Americans frustrate the English because we cannot be pegged from speech alone. In the American culture, an entirely different set of criteria—job, clothing, perceived wealth, vehicle choice, home location and size—establish your credentials. Because I could not be assessed easily in the absence of a British accent, I quickly grew accustomed to routine questioning at the never-ending round of social events, lunches, cocktail parties, dinners, and bashes at the Seaview Yacht Club (very exclusive and membership only), the Mecca for posh villagers.

"So, tell me about your people," was a popular line. "What's your background?" was another. I soon realised it was my superpower not to be pegged by my accent, because of course, an American accent doesn't work that way. Sometimes at a loss at how to peg me, I would hear my all-time favourite line from newly met English acquaintances that found it impossible to glean information about me from my accent. After a bit of chatting, I would hear "Well, in any case, you're quite nice, for an American." (We'll talk more about innate bias later.)

I had truly made in-roads in the village when a debonair old chap at a drinks party, looking the complete landed gentry role in blue blazer with yacht club insignia and white cravat, whispered to me, "Jill, don't have the Greenlies to your house. They aren't P.L.U." I smiled, perplexed, but said nothing.

The Greenlie family were apparently more working class than upper class and were clearly not *People Like Us*. My abhorrence of the innate elitism in his statement once I'd realised what he meant was momentarily quashed by the realisation that *I* was finally considered *P.L.U.* Yippee! I was inside the circle! It didn't cross my mind that after some time, I would see it as a circle I wanted desperately to escape. I felt increasingly like Groucho Marx when he said, "I refuse to join any club that would have me as a member."

After my elation of that first realisation subsided, I noted that the ever-present dichotomy of warmth and reticence about strangers was active. But it was also my good fortune to find pockets of welcome and warmth that touched me deeply, many from the older generation, no longer so interested in status and reaffirming their positioning in society—their positions being secure.

In the house next door to our lovely manor in Seaview lived a retired vicar (a minister in the Anglican community) and his wife Rosalie. In their late 80s and rather rickety, Rosalie never had children of her own.

She was always there to help us, particularly when our children were small, and was exceptionally warm, remarkably open and welcoming; a particular joy for me, with my mother in Colorado. Rosalie's dedication to her neighbours, flowers, lawns, and God were equal, and there were many dark, rainy, late afternoons when I would be popping a cork of fragrant red wine, only to see her through the large bay windows, murky in the cold, wet mist, determinedly mowing her lawns, hunched over in the rain, wearing a huge hat, the rain dribbling off the brim. Her devotion never wavered, rain or shine.

Seaview was a much-adored haven for those who inhabited it; heaven for those who spent their childhood summers on the beach, eating crab ramekins in the tiny front room of the 8-bedroom Seaview Hotel; free to roam round the village barefoot; sailing in the yacht club regattas; drinking Pimm's (a gin-based party punch) in the fading afternoon light on the yacht club's seaside veranda (members only, of course, no riff-raff allowed!), and flitting round the never-ending circle of lawn parties.

For Peter, his history and his heaven were Seaview. For this reason, he wanted to be married in the ancient Anglican Church in the village, with almost the entire village in attendance. This was to be followed with a lavish reception at—where else?—the Seaview Yacht Club.

My first words were **"You want to do what?"** (Yes, I did shout with considerable alarm when Peter lit off this bombshell idea of a second yacht club wedding.) We

37

were already deep into planning a large, white wedding at the swanky Manor House of Ken Caryl Ranch in the Colorado Rockies outside Denver. Peter dropped this bombshell news during a casual conversation on a woodsy walk by the sea one June afternoon.

"Tell me, is there any good reason you can think of why we shouldn't get married twice. Once in Colorado with your people and again in Seaview with mine? It would mean so very much to me, Jill."

Being a level-headed businesswoman, now endowed with a month-long sample of the minefield of English protocol and the shocking revelation that I was completely ignorant about all of it, I said, "Yes, there are loads of reasons why not. How about starting with, I am terrified. How would I put together an invitation list? I don't know anybody here. I've never even been to a wedding in England. I don't know how they work. How can I possibly organize a big wedding in Denver **and** a big wedding in Seaview with only two months to go?" I fretted.

"I'll do it, darling," he simply said. He did not have to tell me again how important this had become to him.

And it was, therefore, decided. He would plan the Seaview wedding and I would manage the Denver wedding. We would have two, one week apart. For most couples, one large wedding usually induces considerable angst, and now there were to be two, on consecutive Saturdays, with a honeymoon in between, within eight days of each other.

Darryl, then-President of Hyatt Hotels and my former boss, generously gave us a week in the presidential suite at any Hyatt Hotel in the world as a wedding gift. We picked Acapulco, Mexico, where we planned to go between the now-inevitable two weddings.

Event planning and all the related events became a kind of schizophrenia—two of everything, except the dress. I'd bought a great dress, or precisely, a dress that held the potential for greatness. I promptly brought it home, tore it apart and was in the process of making modifications, according to my vision of greatness. (Sewing was the sole crafty thing that I could pull off.) The new creation was, of course, white, with a full satin skirt and fitted lace bodice, high necked at the front, with long lace sleeves and a deep "V" shape in the back, almost to the waist. I liked the thrill-factor of seeing the deeply cut back when I turned around after the front view of the high-neckline. Our London flat increasingly looked like a factory floor, with bits of white satin and lace flecked around the place from my sewing, stacks of wedding planning papers on each end of the dining table, one end for the Denver wedding, one end for the Seaview wedding, clock ticking in between.

Late one Sunday afternoon, a month before the weddings, the phone rang. Peter got up from the pile of Seaview wedding papers. It was the Vicar Lowe, from St Peter's Church in Seaview, who had agreed to marry us.

"Bad news I'm afraid, on two fronts," said Vicar Low. "First, I cannot post banns on Jill, which, as I am sure you know, are required for any foreigner to be married on The Island." (We didn't know that).

"I must have the Bishop of The Island approve that Jill is suitable." (Suitable? What does suitable mean?)

"I have made an appointment for you both with Bishop Bucket (the Vicar's boss) for Tuesday at 3:00 PM at his home.

"Secondly, after considerable thought, I have decided I cannot in good conscience marry you in Seaview if you have already been married in America the week before, as you had planned. It is sacrilege to marry twice and makes a mockery of the marriage vows."

The Vicar was adamant that he would not marry us if we had been previously married. I could understand it if the people changed, but marrying the same couple again within a week? What kind of insanity was this? And banns? (What the hell are *banns*?) Are we in the 19th or the 21st Century? *You must be kidding*, I thought. But OK, we'll face the challenge, pay a visit to this Bishop and he'll be supportive, no problem. Feeling bullish, I thought *Bring on the meeting with the Bishop*!

The first issue, the *banns*, was pretty simple. I later learned that *banns* are the proclamation of an intended marriage, posted at least three Sundays prior to the event, to provide an opportunity for objections to be made. We'd simply be ourselves, the Bishop would approve of me, and we'd be off.

The second issue worried us. The invitations were out; Peter had his heart set on it; the plans were made for both ceremonies. We did the only thing we could do. We decided to package the events in a palatable way. We told Vicar Lowe that, considering his comments and our full reverence for this situation, we had "revised" the Denver event, enabling us to be unencumbered entirely with any previous dealings with marriage.

Peter admonished me occasionally when I was relating the story to trusted friends. "Jill, please don't say we 'revised events'. One doesn't lie to a vicar! And the word lie is such a vulgar word. One is simply economical with the truth."

Despite the whole debacle seeming quite funny to me, inside I was a little worried. Could he, would he, really pull the plug on our Seaview wedding? Peter's answer was that he would, he could, and no chances were to be taken. The next weeks had a comical undercurrent with a touch of fear as many friends, already aware of the two events, would see us around the village, at parties or in the Seaview hotel bar, a central gathering place to eat fresh crab ramekins and slug back endless tiny glasses of burgundy. They'd spot us, adopt a sinister grin while looking warily side-to-side for sightings of the vicar in the vicinity. When the coast was clear they would devilishly ask us how the planning for the weddings (capital S) was going, with a smile.

Although we had a good laugh, we were both terrified that the news of the Denver wedding would get back to Vicar Low. Of course, this whole scenario had my family and friends back in the states in hysterics. I never did know exactly what Peter said to the Vicar, but as a master of the double entendre, Peter left him with the impression that the Denver wedding had only been an idea that we were no longer considering and had morphed into a 'party'. It was simply never mentioned thereafter.

Late one afternoon in June, windows open, music blaring, we careened through the leafy lanes of The Island, to the absurdly named, but astonishingly beautiful village of Winkle Street, a row of thatched roof cottages, brimming with flowers on every window ledge. Winkle Street is on the other side of The Island, about 9 miles from Seaview. So, as we drove, we wove through the hedgerows and leafy lanes in anticipation of the meeting with Bishop Bucket to determine if I was "suitable."

I had my sassy and ignorantly confident attitude with me still, ready to be scrutinized by Bishop Bucket. Peter's beloved old Volkswagen Bug screeched up to a geriatric thatched mouse-house, with the ubiquitous greying net curtains billowing out the tiny windows. The doorway was covered with wisteria, the fragrant lavender bunches hung so low we had to bat them away to find the doorbell—the old pull type doorbell with a metal stem you yanked about a foot out of the wall and, as it recedes, elicits a feeble rattle hoping to attract attention. After a couple of pulls, the door creaked open, emitting a musty, atticy smell. Just before the door opened, Peter whispered, "Jill, whatever you say, *please*, don't take the piss," which meant, **be serious**.

The door croaked open, in full anachronistic splendour, displaying Bishop Bucket—all five feet three inches of him, all eighty (at least) years of him. Hunched over, grim-faced, and sporting a worn, floor-length, red robe with a frayed white collar, he wordlessly motioned us to follow him. Peter was told to take a chair, the Bishop pointing a ghostly-white crooked finger toward the corner of the tiny room, where I was instructed to sit, facing him at his desk. I could just see Peter's brow lift in worried angst but with a touch of warning out of the corner of his eye as I lowered down onto the edge of my chair. A billow of dust engulfed me post-perch, camouflaging a snort and a giggle from me. I swallowed them both.

"So, Miss Bausch."

"Yes, Bishop?" smiling sweetly.

"I understand you wish to marry Mr. Brook."

"Yes, Bishop."

"Why?"

Unprepared for this question, I stammered, "Ah, ah, well, Bishop, we are very well suited and we love each other." Then, thinking I would get an extra point with the Bishop, I added, "And we are culturally diverse enough to learn a great deal from one another." This seemed to please him.

"Do you intend to have children?"

"Yes, sir," I said, knowing full well that Peter and I had never finalized our discussions on this topic.

"Good, this is God's will."

"Yes, sir."

A few more general inquiries were floated about my background (of course), my people (of course) my faith, my bloodlines, my devotion to England, Great Britain, and all the people of the British Isles. I subserviently responded to all in the affirmative. I was true to my future husband, to glorious England, to The Queen and all her subjects. The Bishop simply emitted the occasional, "hmmmmmmm," seeming satisfied, to which I thought, *This is a piece of cake. I am suitable!* Bishop Bucket then leaned his miniature frame toward me over his dusty desk and said, "Vicar Low in Seaview informs me that Peter and his family have a rich history with the Anglican Church in Seaview, as I am sure you know."

"Yes, Bishop."

"Your background and intention seem suitable for him."

This seemed a preposterous statement from the bishop, since Peter had no such history, and had not uttered a peep, nor was he asked to throughout the proceedings. But I kept quiet since it was going so well and resisted my overwhelming temptation to say, "How the heck would you know, exactly?" This would be precisely what Peter would call *taking the piss.*

The bishop continued, "The only formality left is for me to know which Diocese you belong to in America. It is required that you are affiliated with an appropriate diocese for me to give my approval to post the banns. The banns will then be posted for a month prior to your wedding, and if there are no objections from the islanders, you may proceed."

An expletive entered my mind and, fortunately, remained there alone. Diocese? What Diocese? He obviously can't tell I'm a pagan, even a heathen. But how am I going to get out of this? Peter was looking distinctly green, brows lowered to a scowling frown. The bishop reached to his left and pulled down a gigantic book with gold Latin lettering on its worn leather cover. My head raced as I thought: This midget octogenarian has the power to pull the plug on our future! What can I do? Another blanket of dust wafted out and settled when he opened the Big Book of Worldwide Dioceses.

"So, which is it?" he asked, eyes down scouring the pages for the US listings.

"Well Bishop, you know that the Anglican Church is not very prevalent in the USA."

I was biding time, panicking, trying to think of a way out.

"I know, child," he said casting spurious looks at both Peter and me. Then, sounding exasperated, "but we have affiliates. Which is yours?"

"Ah, well, Bishop, it's the, ah, the Diocese of Pittsford."

I spat out the name of the small town in Upstate New York where I grew up. I was cornered like a rat.

"Hmmmmm," grunted Bishop Buckett, "that doesn't seem to be listed," furiously scanning his pages.

"Oh, Bishop," I fibbed through clenched teeth, "It's a new diocese, just set up a few years ago. Unless your book has been updated, it won't be listed yet."

Something told me that the big book of Dioceses was updated only about once a century. At this point, I thought Peter was about to gag over the bishop's dusty carpet, his eyes out on stalks. We were both holding our breath. There was an interminable moment of silence and then, Bishop Buckett erupted, "Wonderful!" while slapping the filthy book closed with a thud. "That's that, then. Congratulations!"

And so, I was immortalized, for a month anyway, on a 12-inch by 12-inch poster, as "Spinster, Jill Bausch," affixed to every village church news board and telephone pole throughout The Island, just waiting for Bishop Bucket to ring us with reams of protests about my intentions to marry one of The Island's own sons. But incredibly, he never rang. I will always wonder what Vicar Lowe thought when he saw my very tan back in the dress as we turned and walked back down the aisle at wedding number two.

It was here that I learned the value of being my authentic self, even when a bit of packaging is called for so that I can protect my corner.

IMPOSTER SYNDROME

In Chapter One, I said, "If you don't feel confident, imagine a role model, someone you admire, role play in your head how they would handle" a situation that overwhelmed you. "How would they hold themselves, look, and speak? What would they wear? Mirror them. … You can, and will, with the right practice, become what you can only now pretend to be."

I'm not suggesting that you lie or in any way deceive co-workers, family, or friends. Life is a learning process and the best learning comes through active practice. Even when you don't feel confident, you can act as if you do. Over time, you will gain the confidence you feel, and the act becomes the reality.

As this process unfolds, you'll probably feel **fear**—you wouldn't be human if you didn't. This is "imposter syndrome", a subconscious use of negative behaviours to cover up some internal (subconscious) fear. In this case, I believe the fear is threefold:

- Fear of not being able to do what you've set out to do
- Fear that others will find out that you're somehow not up to the job
- A lack of confidence that comes from society's attitudes toward women

This fear may generate self-doubt:

- "What happens when someone else figures out that I'm not up to it?"

- "Am I going to lose face, lose my job, not be what I want to be?"
- "Will I be seen as overbearing, aggressive and too tough?"

This doubt can lead to behaviours that feed the self-doubt:

- Diminishing or dismissing compliments
- Talking down what you've accomplished
- Caring too much about what others think of me
- Declining needed help because your fear says, "I have to do it on my own"
- Constantly comparing yourself to others and coming up (in your own mind) short

All research shows that imposter syndrome is very common, and, as we said earlier, far more so in women than in men. I think it comes in part from our upbringing. The standards women are expected to keep, formed by family or societal pressures and reflected in the workplace, make women far less secure in themselves. Most men are quick to say, "I don't know this, but I can figure it out." That's another societal norm, a standard attitude imposed on men for generations: You stand on your own two feet and get the job done! And, they do. They will step up and ask to be selected for a role when they may have far fewer skills than the women competing, but much higher confidence.

Women are taught to spend so much time trying to meet the expectations of us as a "supportive" friend, girlfriend, mother, wife, partner, worker, manager, that we can forget we're having to learn and relearn things in a world that's not only constantly changing, but in which changes are constantly accelerating.

Women sometimes don't rise to the level of our innate ability because our society still puts this pressure on us. All this feeds imposter syndrome to the point where it can spiral out of control to become a paralyzing fear, even for some of the most senior, successful professional women.

AUTHENTICITY

Let me be perfectly clear on this point, I'm not suggesting **being a fake**. "Fake it 'til you make it" is a commonly-used and well understood phrase. It means **acting** the part until you **learn** the part. You can't permanently fake who you are, people will eventually figure you out. More important, you'll know you're faking it and it'll blow your self-confidence, making imposter syndrome worse. You end up thinking, "How long can I fake this? This isn't really who I am."

The most effective response to imposter syndrome lies in aligning your external and internal selves.

After discussing this concept with many people, I've concluded that "authenticity," in this usage, is "being true to who you are." That is the simplest expression I know to prevent imposter syndrome from derailing your success.

In Chapter One, I also used an example—a board room with 20 people, just one or two of them women. I said you may wonder, "Are we supposed to be here?"

I responded, "Yes. ... Because you're there. ... You [convinced] a group of selectors ... that you're the right person for that job."

That's the authentic you, the one chosen because she was qualified. You might be afraid the selectors were wrong. That's perfectly normal, everybody feels that way at some point in life.

If you're not as confident as you want to be, walk the talk. Do the job, mirror your role models, behave and think as though you've been confident all your life. John Wayne, the American cowboy film star, famously said, "Courage is being scared to death, but saddling up anyway." Scared people have "saddled up" in millions of situations and grown into the person the situation demanded. Is there some reason you absolutely can't do the same?

So, how do you know that you're doing it right?

There is an external you—the face you present to the world, and an internal you—the face you present only to yourself and trusted, intimate friends. **Authenticity is the alignment of the two.** Does your external self—your actions, conversations, decisions—align with your internal self—your values, ethics, priorities? At the end of the day:

- Are you happy with what you said in that meeting?
- Are you satisfied with how you treated that co-worker?

- Did you answer a question with, "I don't know, let me get back to you," or, "We need to check with another department"?
- Did you say, "I can't do that, do we have someone more experienced who can take that on?"

If so, you're on the right track. But don't get too comfortable, success breeds promotion, and there's a landmine hiding around that corner.

CIRCUMVENTING THE PETER PRINCIPLE

Way back in 1969, Dr. Laurence Peter and Raymond Hull published *The Peter Principle* as something of a satire on business management. "The Peter Principle" states that people in any hierarchy tend to rise to "a level of respective incompetence."

It works like this: XYZ Company takes John Doe, a skilled engineer, and makes him an engineering supervisor. John does very well, so the executives promote him to engineering manager. John does moderately well and the executives promote him to general manager. John is now faced with mostly non-engineering tasks and he doesn't do well. He has reached his level of "incompetence"—his skill set no longer matches his role. He's been given responsibilities he was never trained to handle, so he appears to be *incompetent*, when, in fact, he is simply *unschooled*—and, possibly, *untalented*. Had the company provided a management training program, John may have discovered he just doesn't have what it takes to deal with the non-engineering challenges and stayed happy as a supervisor or manager. The company failed to understand that skills which create success in one area don't automatically translate to success in all areas.

I had a potential Peter imposter syndrome incident when I was asked to become CEO of Futures Group Europe. At first, I declined. I told my future boss, Robert, the Chairman of the Board, "No, thank you. I'm a mom of a three- and a five-year-old. I'm not missing their rugby games and their ballet recitals and special life moments."

He replied, "I've never missed a baseball game. (He lived in America.) You don't ever have to miss those moments. You just have to get the work done."

I then accepted the challenge but soon realized that every CEO with whom I interacted had a master's degree. I also heard some comments about me, "Oh, I can't believe she got the job, she doesn't even have a master's."

Two significant issues now arose which could've sunk my chances of success:

- There's a whole bank of knowledge I didn't have about sexual and reproductive health and population.
- There's a lack of credentials which would've led to a credibility gap between me and my professional peers.

I was neck deep in an imposter syndrome situation.

So, I went back to Robert, who was a great mentor. He said, "You do need a master's, for your own self-confidence and for credibility in the field. We'll give you the paid time off you'll need to take the classes, as long as you make up for the work at other times. So, go get it if you're willing to do it."

The company had actually taken a huge risk, hiring someone without the expected degree. I guess they just had a lot of faith in me, but how would we fit it all in? I say "we" because I had a husband and two small children and this would affect them, also. We came up with a plan and I went to the London School of Economics. I did take time off work for classes and caught up at night and on the weekends. I took two years to complete an LSE master's course that usually required one, but I learned a lot that was essential to the job I was doing.

That mentoring erased the "imposter syndrome" for me and prevented me from being "Peter-ed." The comments disappeared because, in that world, credentials mean a lot.

Was this the best way? For me, in that situation, it was, absolutely. You have to judge your situation, weigh the positives and negatives, assess the costs and benefits, then come up with a plan and execute it. I'm a big believer in brain food—not every day, that would overwhelm us and we'd never fit it all in—but regularly. Especially in light of the many changes happening in almost every part of life and culture these days, you have to be prepared for what's on the horizon and what's over it. The Master's degree I took was in

Population and International Development, and it was the right brain-food for me at that time.

(There's a flip side to this coin. When you're the senior person with up-and-coming juniors, you should be willing to give others the same trust and opportunities you were given. I'd like to discuss that in depth, but that's another whole book.)

As we rise from technician (for lack of a better term) to supervisor, then manager, then executive, we need to add personnel management, financial, legal, and other skills. Those are the easy part. There are good schools all over the world that provide solid technical training. Almost anyone can understand these disciplines well enough to understand how these factors affect their organisation. The real challenge has always been to develop strategic thinking, planning, and decision-making skills and, of course, emotional intelligence. These separate the technician from the executive. To develop those new skills, coaching and mentoring are vital. But they are very different inputs.

COACHING

Coaching is focused on an organisation's key assets, its people, both as individuals and as team members. A coach works with you, using your own agenda to enable you to break through to new ways of looking at your world—called "thinking outside the box" or "lateral thinking." The coach uses specialized techniques to unleash your internal potential and helps you identify your skills and talents—your "toolbox"—and hone those tools to peak performance. Coaching supports you in finding your own solutions, asking questions like, "How do you think you could look at it differently?" or, "How would you feel if you did that or this?"

Most senior professionals in business today have a coach and know their value. They wouldn't be able to navigate the "bumps in the road" so skillfully or to improve without their coach.

I'll give one quick example: Your "demeanor" is how you carry yourself, how you appear to others. Back in the hotel business I used to teach people how to behave on camera—TV and radio news interviews, talks shows, podcasts, and other media. (Such invitations get more frequent as you become a recognized expert or thought leader in your field.) During my training to do this work, they also interviewed me on video. Viewing it afterwards, I saw a whole lot of things that I didn't realize I was doing. I spoke too fast. I wiggled my leg. Women also tend to lean their heads to the side. You almost never see men do that but watch for it, you'll see us do it a lot. It's a common body language response to lack of confidence.

These are distracting habits which, subconsciously, reduce credibility. I never knew I fell into that same trap and wouldn't ever have noticed them if an external party had not pointed out what I was doing.

Coaching is a reality check, a chance for someone who'll look at you without bias and tell you the truth about how well you listen, how clearly you speak, how well you conduct a meeting and a hundred other topics. If you trust your coaches, take their lessons to heart, and let experience prove them right. Life gets so much easier.

While you're at it, don't be afraid of failure. It's a fundamental part of the human experience. Henry Ford once said, "Failure is only the opportunity to begin again more intelligently." Many have attested that they learn more from their failures than from their successes. I firmly believe you can always get something out of failure, even if it's just that you need additional training in this or that skill. More on making failure work for you in a later chapter.

MENTORING

Mentoring is external guidance and advice from a senior level source, one with more experience—more "stripes"—in a similar business sector. In essence, a suitable mentor has "been there, done that." If the protégé asks, "What would you do?" The mentor may respond, "Well, when I was in that job, I did this." The protégé can use that example as a starting point for their decisions. Mentors aren't giving directions, but trying to stimulate your own ideas with experiences from their own career or the experience of colleagues in similar situations:

- "Have you thought about the X-Y-Z process?"
- "Why don't you do 1, 2, and 3 and see if that works?"

By the way, you can be mentored by people long dead. Sir Isaac Newton famously said, "If I have seen farther, it is by standing on the shoulders of giants." He built on centuries of knowledge compiled by previous mathematicians. Someone once joked that we study history so we don't repeat their mistakes, freeing us up to make new mistakes of our own.

According to a recent article in *Business News Daily*[5]:

"Anyone looking for a mentor should keep these three things in mind:

- "Define what you want out of your career and what you need to learn to get there."
- "Approach a mentor relationship as if it's a business friendship – be casual and friendly."
- "Start with your own professional network. We often already have mentors who provide advice in various ways, and all it takes is a little effort from us to grow that connection into an ongoing relationship."

Many sources discuss multiple values of mentoring:

- The mentor/protégé relationship is a "safe space." Like a parent, faith leader, or medical professional, challenges can be discussed in absolute privacy. Mentoring must be impartial, free of bias or office politics.
- Privacy breeds transparency. With a mentor outside your company, you can openly discuss

---

[5] Matt D'Angelo, "How to Find a Mentor," *BusinessNewsDaily. com*, Waltham, MA: *Business News Daily*, 2021. https://www. businessnewsdaily.com/6248-how-to-find-mentor.html, accessed 9 June 2022.

personal challenges related to or deriving from the job.

- Good mentors provide honest, unbiased feedback and new perspectives.
- Good mentors will introduce you to others, expanding your professional network, opening opportunities for discussion, cooperation, future employment (yours in their organization or them in yours), and other mutually beneficial ventures.
- Open, frank discussions can reboot creative thought and inspire innovation.

Mentoring, I should add, can also be a formal program within an organization. Executives can assist supervisors/managers in understanding and implementing the organization's goals "in the company way" and adjusting to the company culture. That's different from the professional mentoring I just described, but can also be valuable in preparing junior leaders for more senior roles.

PRACTICAL FACTORS

Some companies still don't understand the Peter Principle and it remains a problem. When you're offered a promotion or new job, you have to accept or decline it based on facts. Most women want the added responsibility and influence, as well as the prestige and pay increase that accompany a promotion. On the flip side, some people just want to do what they do because they love doing it and don't want the added responsibility, time commitment or stress. Both are perfectly legitimate choices.

Those who want to step upward have to take a serious look at what they know and what they don't know, in terms of what that new job requires. They need to ask themselves hard questions and give themselves honest reactions:

- Do I know enough to fulfill all the requirements of that new position?
- If I don't know, can I learn?
- If I can learn, do I want to learn?
- If you don't want to learn, you should decline the promotion.

Get this conversation with yourself right, then set yourself up with the right coaches and mentors and you've set yourself up with the best odds for success. You'll minimize imposter syndrome and probably avoid the Peter Principle.

Stepping up from the imposter to the authentic character is a challenge for many women. It means overcoming generations of false expectations and upbringing. Overcoming those cultural biases requires an understanding of who you really are. It aligns those inner values with your outer persona. Get the coaching that develops your lateral thinking, and the mentoring that allows you to stand on the shoulders of those who've gone before.

CHAPTER 4

YOUR NOT-TO-DO LIST IS YOUR BFF

The vision that you glorify in your mind, the ideal that you enthrone in your heart, this you will build your life by, and this you will become.

—James Allen, *As A Man Thinketh*

To succeed in life, you need three things: a wishbone, a backbone, and a funny bone.

—Reba McEntire (attributed)

INTRODUCTION — WOMEN SUFFERING WITH IMPOSTER SYNDROME

To continue: People who doubt their abilities, to the point they feel like a fraud, suffer from "imposter syndrome."

This disability disproportionately affects high-achieving people, many of whom find it difficult to accept their accomplishments. As we know, it also disproportionately affects women over men.

As a talent management specialist, a head-hunter for international organisations, and an executive coach, I come across countless exceptionally senior and highly-skilled women who suffer with the fear they'll be "found out." What does that even mean?

It means that, deep down, they really don't believe they deserve the job they have. They don't believe they have the skills that others believe they have. They believe they are where they are by some stroke of luck or wish or that it was a mistake that put them in top leadership positions around the world. Notice, not they "don't **deserve** the job" but they "don't **believe they deserve** the job." There's a difference. Also, as already noted, they didn't just walk in and take over, they were **selected** by people specifically charged to hire the best qualified candidates for those positions. These women are **not** where they are by mistake or because of some accident, yet many women continue to doubt themselves.

I spoke to a very senior woman at Interpol, the International Criminal Police Organization, a law enforcement agency operating in 195 member countries. She was considering a move to another high-profile role and wanted my advice on her interview technique. She had misgivings about being seen as a role model for younger women coming up through the ranks. She sincerely wanted to help them but thought that if she was her authentic, firm, straight-talking self, she'd appear pushy and aggressive. She asked about tools to deliver her message authentically but without risking criticism for her strength.

How is it that, saying exactly the same words, we see a man as **assertive** but a woman as **aggressive**? How is it that we see an **aggressive male** as a positive but an **aggressive female** as a negative? This woman had doubted herself for years, even though she rose consistently through the ranks in international roles. She, by then, had held several senior positions and had a solid record of success in those jobs. That's why she kept getting senior jobs. Yet, in spite of all that, she suffered imposter syndrome.

In another case, I lead the search for the Assistant Secretary General of a large United Nations agency. SRI Executive, the firm where I work, and other executive search agencies, employ global research teams specifically to look for people with exceptional reputations and exceptional digital footprints. We keep them on our radar to consider when these important leadership roles come open. With a research team member as my number two for every search I lead, we carefully research candidates' credentials. We go through numerous assessments and, if they finally get to an interview with me, they've passed every test we can devise to be certain they're qualified for that post.

In this case, aware of its gender and diversity position, the UN hierarchy felt the need to have a woman from the global south. Frankly, too many of the most influential roles in the world are held by males from the global north, so, we're often asked to seek candidates whose viewpoints will bring some measure of balance to the discussion. While there is arguably a sort of inverted bias in this approach, it is nonetheless, widespread.

When my team brought me the list of final candidates— five women—for this role, each one had remarkable credentials. However, when I spoke to them, three said they weren't certain they had the full credentials for the role and the other two said they wanted to get more experience before they went for a role that substantial. Why were they hesitant? Imposter syndrome. Were they afraid of not getting the role and having to live with the repercussions of coming in second best (which, in this arena, would actually have been an achievement to be proud of)? Or did they fear getting the job and not feeling credible?

EXPECTATIONS OR THE LACK THEREOF

In the website announcement for his new book, *The Expectation Effect*, David Robson argues for the power of the mind in personal and professional success:

- People who believe ageing brings wisdom live longer.
- Lucky charms really do improve an athlete's performance.
- Reappraising stress as energising increases your creativity under pressure.
- Cultivating an indulgent attitude to food helps you lose weight.
- Taking a placebo, even when you know it is a placebo, can still improve your health.

Robson continues: "Of course, you can't just think yourself thinner, happier or fitter, but using this book you can *reframe* many different facets of your life, and in so doing, start real psychological, physiological and behavioural change. These easy-to-use skills will help you on your way to becoming the person you want to be, living the life you want to live."[6]

I wonder if, somehow, men naturally understand this, but women somehow find this more difficult through the upbringing and norms that society teaches them. The ideas Robson puts forward aren't new. A generation ago, salesman, author, and motivational speaker, the late Zig Zigler frequently said, "It's your attitude, not your aptitude, that determines your altitude." Over a century ago, James Allen's famous *As A Man Thinketh* included the quote that leads this chapter.

Intellectually, we understand this concept. It's as simple as anything you'll ever hear. But we don't always feel it deep in our hearts and our psyches, so it isn't reflected in our attitude about ourselves and our resulting self-confidence and behaviour. Men expect success, as if bred to it, which brings a whole different set of mental health challenges when they don't succeed, but that is for someone else's book.

Women—even the very talented, highly-experienced women I have the privilege of working with—seem to have a significant lack of success expectation and increased insecurity in dealing with the success they do achieve. So, what do we do about it?

---

[6] David Robson, "The Expectation Effect," *DavidRobson.me*, New York City: Henry Holt & Co., 2022. https://davidrobson.me/books/the-expectation-effect/, accessed 17 June 2022.

BACKGROUND

Let me start with some personal history: I already mentioned that I received my undergraduate degree in the United States, then my master's degree at London School of Economics, to get added professional credentials, in the late 1990s.

Some years later, my family spent time in Burkina Faso for my husband's work, followed by an assignment in France. I left my own position, needing a sabbatical, and we relocated to West Africa. During that time, I started thinking, "I need to listen better. There's something I'm good at here, but I'm not really sure how to package it." When I was a CEO, many people told me, "You're a really good boss." Mentally, I responded, "Oh, am I? Okay, thank you." But I couldn't say why I was a good boss. And I didn't ask. I was teaching Master's Degree behavioural economics classes at the University of Denver before the move and I got more interested in the psychological aspects of leadership and more interested in human behaviours generally. This was the beginning of the Not-To-Do list idea. I thought, "I'm going to take myself off and learn to be an executive coach, and get certified."

I chose the Academy of Executive Coaching in London and got my certification. Among other things, they focused on listening, hearing, and asking questions in place of being instructive or directive. This was a great help in changing my style and avoiding bad habits, converting thinking into doing, turning directive advice into probing questions to help others find their own way to a solution or improvement they are seeking.

At the same time during my coaching courses, we discussed things that keep people back from the success they're really capable of achieving. It's been said that depression is debilitating and anxiety is motivating. Generally, I agree, though I wouldn't say it's always true. Anxiety or depression, as well as overwork, unrealistic expectations, and other stresses can cause women to feed into imposter syndrome. How do we deal with those stresses?

I was starting to build a toolbox full of strategies people use to do just that:

There's the **replay** method, where you sit down and interview yourself, "That outcome wasn't what I was after. How could I replay it if I could do it again? How will I replay it if something similar ever comes up?"

There's also **courtroom** method, where you put your fears on trial, "I feel anxious about a deliverable or a relationship with somebody, but where are the facts? Where's the evidence? Am I worrying because there's a problem or because I think something some problem might arise?" In fact, people frequently worry about things that aren't happening, where there are no facts to support that the worry will happen, and, 99 percent of the time, they never do happen. Are you creating a narrative that does not factually exist, but is at the heart of it what you fear will happen?

There are also simple yet powerful tools—things like meditation, watching your diet, and generally staying healthy, which make your body better able to deal with stress. These have a positive physical as well as mental-emotional effect.

These and many other tools in the box, are valuable but, along the way, I noticed that, in my training, we were spending our time discussing what we *should* do. At some point, I started asking myself, why aren't we spending time discussing what we *shouldn't do* or *don't need to do*? Or, even, what we don't need to do *now*?

For me, the coaching experience was mostly about each person finding their own form and format. In other words, what works for you? I concluded that, for me at least, what I didn't do was just as important a revelation as what I did need and want to do.

A TOOL FOR SELF-MANAGEMENT

A quick, obvious disclaimer: No system is perfect; no solution works for every problem. The Not-To-Do list isn't the answer to every challenge. It's one of many tools available to help you manage yourself and your activities, to help you set yourself up for success. The Not-To-Do list idea is an extension of something I wrote about in the introduction to this book:

> If you don't feel confident, imagine a role model, someone you admire. Roleplay in your head how they would handle it. How would they hold themselves, look, and speak? What would they wear? Mirror them. I'm often asked if it's possible to teach confidence. Yes; if you mirror it enough, it becomes a habit. While this habit develops, you may fear being exposed as

a fraud. If you do, you may have what is called "imposter syndrome." ... You can, and will, with the right mentoring and practice, become what you can only now pretend to be.

That's why teaching about success includes a lot of time on what to do to achieve it. This book asks what should be the twin question: What must we *not-do* to achieve success? It was written to help you overcome ineffective habits and replace them with effective habits. Saying no to when it's warranted is one of those effective habits. That's the "backbone" part of what Reba McEntire meant in the quote attributed to her at the start of this chapter.

For example, when asked to take on a new project, thinking, "If I say no, will people assume I can't do it?" is a bad habit. You can't be successful at making decisions based on what other people think of you. You want a good reputation, but establishing boundaries, which we discussed a little in a previous chapter, is another keystone of success. The Not-To-Do list is, partly, that boundary.

The position you hold in an organization—your seniority by job or experience—generally determines how often and to whom you can say, "No," to and get away with it. You need to consider that and several other factors:

- "Do I want to do that or not?" If I want to do it, it's a slam-dunk no-brainer. That said, there are external factors that can prevent you: Does your workload allow you to take on a new project? Do you have or can you acquire the skill set and other resources necessary to complete the project? Are there non-project related factors that could preclude success? If all the answers are favorable, I say, "Great, let's talk about how we're going to get it done."

- If I'm hesitant about it, I might say, "What is it you want from me? Do you want me to listen to you? Do you want inputs from me? Do you want me to help you brainstorm how to complete this? Do you want to hand it over to someone else? What is it you feel you need?"

- If I don't think I'm the person for the project, I might say, "What, specifically, do you need? Maybe I'm not the best person to do this, because this isn't in my area of expertise or I can't fit it into my workload right now." You can always add ideas on how to do it or who to talk to, without committing yourself to participate.

I prefer to ask questions instead of just saying, "No, I'm not doing it." Once I have a full picture of the project, that is, once I have **listened to** whoever proposed the project—given them the professional respect and courtesy they deserve—I can make an informed decision. I also encourage the requester by giving them the satisfaction of knowing I listened and considered and decided yes or no based on all the facts. Anyone who expects more than that has unreasonable expectations. (And, sadly, there are plenty of those people in the world.) Find phrases that are straightforward, polite, but clearly mean no, and are still authentically you. For example, "I'd like to help but my workload won't allow it right now" or "You might find someone more suitable than me to do this because I can't fit it in."

MAKING A NOT-TO-DO LIST

People are so pressured by their To-Do lists that they often don't properly consider priorities. Skewed priorities are among the best ways to be professionally insecure or burnt out, and lower the quality of your output on the work and home fronts.

THE IDEA

Get out your To-Do list and move some items to a Not-To-Do list.

- Consider each item: Does it have to be done **now** or **today**? If not, put it on today's Not-To-Do list.
- Say no to items that aren't vital to do today. Use your practiced phrasing that gets the message across in a way that leaves you feeling comfortable, such as, "I'd like to help you with that, but I can't fit it in just now."
- Remember to say no to yourself, as well as to others. Imagine you were paying someone else to do things you're planning to do. Imagine you're billing yourself for doing all the small things that keep you in the weeds and away from doing the important things. In either of those scenarios, would the effort be worth the money? How much money would you lose by wasting time on those items?
- Finally, having sifted through and shortened the To-Do list, relentlessly attack it!

THE METHOD

For me, there are two sides to this coin—behaviour and tasks.

I make lists. I've got lists on my phone and sticky notes all over my desk, but I don't get up every morning and create To-Do and Not-To-Do lists for each day. I make those decisions in my head the night before.

I set some priorities on those lists based on behaviours. I tell myself:

- "These are some of my weaker areas. Don't over-dwell on these things. Get help when needed."
- "Don't overthink things, especially the smaller things."
- "Don't ruminate on issues or worry about things, just address them, and if you need to fix them, fix them."

I set other priorities on the lists based on tasks:

- "I don't like doing this, so let's get it out of the way."
- "Is this task better suited to another team member?"
- "Can I delegate this to another team member so I can focus on things I have to do myself?"
- "Would this task be a good training or mentoring exercise for another team member?"

As a headhunter, our organization has teams all over the world and different people to support me on each project or piece of leadership work. It's not that I have one assistant and I can say, "Okay, you do that." I have seven or eight assistants at any time. I have to balance their workloads, keep them progressing, build on strengths and strengthen weaknesses, ensure they are learning and growing, feel included, and generally be the team leader. I have to think through, "What's my function on this project?" Mostly, I am the client-facing person. I keep the client feeling they are in a safe pair of hands. I talk to the hiring research teams every day, teach them about a new sector, or steer them in the right direction to understand the roles. I get them to understand the nuances of every detail of a position, and do final interviews before submitting a candidate. I'm a role model when we are facing a client. The assistants do the research and the paperwork.

As I split these lists in my head, I can also decide "I don't have to do that, maybe ever!" It may mean I don't have to do that now, or I don't have to do that ever, but I've then created a Not-To-Do-Ever list. There are benefits that come with a substantial career investment, so I sometimes ask myself, "What don't I need to spend my time on?" and make delegation decisions. I can give many tasks to my co-lead, to an assistant, or to some other team member on any given headhunting project. Sometimes, however, the task is mine and mine alone. No one else can coach someone who's hired me to coach them. We have clients who want me to lead calls and conversations, and relationships matter more than anything. Knowing the difference makes managing professional life far simpler and more successful.

Another important point is exemplified here: Priorities change, often minute-by-minute! (You know this.) Some things, of course, have to be done on a specific schedule, regardless of any other considerations. Excluding emergencies, most of your regular, professional tasks never come as a surprise. They are scheduled far in advance. That makes them very simple. When the scheduled tasks come due, they shoot to the head of the priority list. They get done and then it's back to the Not-To-Do until the schedule comes around again.

As I develop those lists, division of labour must be considered. Sometimes, if it needs to be done by close-of-business day, I just do it. At other times, I decide it should be done by my partner or my assistant. In our home, we do have a division of labour and sometimes we plan it, but sometimes, it's just divided up naturally, one of us sees a need and does it. That should also happen in the office. Taking the initiative is a great habit in any organization, especially among junior team members who want to become senior members.

When I decide another team member should do something for me, or I'm on the fence about it, I ask, "Do you have time for this?" The leader needs to be respectful of subordinates' time, and I've always found that very motivating, especially to the more junior team members. It's nothing more than professional courtesy and respect. I was so happy when Outlook created their <Send Later> button. If I'm working late or on the weekend, I can write emails without ruining anybody's time off. I just set the program to send them out the next business day at seven o'clock and we're ready to go when we get to work. I don't want the junior people to feel they have to respond on a weekend, just because that is the time I decided to catch up on work.

The goal of all this is simply to get the job done as well as it can be and be respectful of others at the same time. We want our people to be happy because when they are, they do their best work. (You know this, too.) Since COVID struck, as remote work has risen (and I expect it will continue to increase as an alternative), the beginning and ending of the work day has become much more flexible for many people. I've been working from home for 20 years now, so I'm pretty good about saying, "It's six o'clock or six thirty, I'm shutting it down." Some people aren't so good at it yet and do need to be encouraged to set boundaries. I don't want to be that leader who expects them to be looking at and responding to emails in their off time. I want to be a role model who respects the work/life balance and I want you to be that, too.

THE RESULT

How do you know you're doing it right—that your Not-To-Do list is effective? In our organization, we have a formal, online system of evaluation. I assess team members and they give me feedback on how each headhunting process went. With the United Nations and other international organisations, we really hope projects don't take more than six months, but it can take a year to search, find, negotiate, and place a high-level person. Whenever it's completed, I have to rank the people working with me on a number of different items: How did they do? What could they do better? I tell them what I would like them to do **more of** or **less of** on the next project. I like to keep it simple, asking them for more of this, less of that. For their appraisal of me, I ask them, "What would you like me to do more of? What would you like me to do less of?" That's an easy and safe way to give me feedback without feeling that they've been critical of the boss. We've been doing it this way for some time and we feel very good about the results. By the way, I generally get the same comments over and over again on what I should do less of or more of, which is interesting. And I do try to do less or more of those things. I really listen. I try to modify my behaviour based on what I've heard. You'll read a lot more about listening a bit later in this book.

CONCLUSION

In leadership and leadership education, what we do is important and what we don't do is equally important. These practices are vital in developing the positive habits that create our pathway to success, avoiding negative habits that hinder success and, ultimately, assist us in growing to be the best leaders and professionals that we can be.

The Not-To-Do list is a tool of self- and team-management that can be very valuable in relieving stress. Anxiety, depression, overwork, unrealistic expectations, and other stresses can cause women to fall into imposter syndrome.

Creating a Not-To-Do list, to complement your To-Do list, is also a proactive decision-making practice that helps you divide responsibilities among your team, avoid doing work that others should do, focus on work that you must do, and manage team members' activities so that each works, but doesn't overwork, to give you their best efforts.

CHAPTER 5

LISTENING

Some of my best communication has come from listening.

—Corina Thurston

INTRODUCTION — LISTENING TO MYSELF

21 DECEMBER 1988

I sat that day in my office at Marriott Headquarters on Piccadilly Square in London, getting acquainted and discussing business with my new boss, who'd arrived a few days before on his first trip to England from the United States. He told me that his wife and children were concerned about his need to travel internationally in his new job, how close they were as a family, and how much he missed them. That same day, we both boarded planes—him on a flight to return home to the US; I on a flight for a long-planned holiday in Australia, spending Christmas with my husband. When I landed in Sydney, I saw the news: My boss's flight, Pan American 103, blew up over Lockerbie, Scotland, victim of a terrorist bomb. The flight crew of 16, all 243 passengers, and 11 residents of that small, peaceful town, died horribly.

I descended into a spiral of fear about the world, with no reserves of bravery. I felt like my life was on a precipice, just as my boss' unknowingly had been, liable to be ended at any moment, for no reason I could control. I had to choose to hide or choose to be brave.

Days and weeks passed. Back in London, still jittery, I saw a counsellor, and we talked about how scary the world felt and I tried to make sense of my fear. I couldn't live in fear because that isn't a life. I knew this instinctively, my mind kept saying it, but the rest of me wasn't listening. I realized that I had to learn to listen to what my mind was saying. Of course, I also needed to listen to others and take reasonable precautions where potential threats were known. That's just common sense. But, at my core, I needed to listen to **me**, to use my free will and choose to face my life, and all its uncertainties, with courage, instead of living in fear over what might never happen.

Over time, I made that final choice for bravery. I decided that I would listen to myself, make decisions with courage and wisdom—but without fear—and to help others do the same, however I could.

Some Years Later

I was in Burkina Faso and the monsoons hit. The city of Ouagadougou became one vast mud pit. In this area, monsoons come after what are called the Harmattan winds, sandstorms of western Africa like tornadoes of pure grit. They blinded those who couldn't take cover fast enough. They filled our screened porch with inches of sand almost daily. The grit seeped through the same cracks in the house that the giant geckos used to sneak in and gather in our rafters. (Those creepy lizards kept me up at night with their scrambling around under the roof in the grit.)

We offered to drive our cook, Daniel, to his home on the outskirts of this heaving mud pit, one of many areas housing Ouagadougou's million destitute people. I had, by then, worked many years in international development and travelled through some of the poorest places on earth. Living in Ouagadougou, however, was still an eye-opener. The combination of the heat (frequently topping 40° Celsius/104° Fahrenheit), the Harmattan sandstorms, the rain, the poverty, and the language barrier (they only speak French or Arabic. At the time, I spoke neither), were overwhelming to live with. We put Daniel, a lovely, ageing Burkinabe father of seven, in our clapped-out aid worker's 4-wheel drive SUV and drove through (literally) feet of mud to his home—a mud hut. Daniel's little motorbike would never have gotten him home though the miles of long, slippery mud tracks.

Following his directions, we travelled endless off-the-beaten mud paths and sludgy side roads, finally arriving at a circle of huts (mud, of course) melting under the monsoon deluge. Daniel's large family was gathered around the huts, waiting for their patriarch to return. Many of them were crying. When you live in a mud hut with few material possessions, watching your home disappear before your eyes is a new kind of heart-wrenching experience.

We asked Daniel if we could bring his large family back to our house. Our house was full of sand from the Harmattans but, at least, it was on concrete foundations, had running water, and shelter from the sand and rains. Daniel's pride would not let him say yes. About 55, I think, he was old by their standards, and had lived through this many, many times before, maybe every year of his life. As patriarch of that family, he firmly thanked us but decided they would be best staying home. I really listened to him—not just the words, but the thoughts and emotions behind the words, and I watched the faces of his family, who trusted him without question. Earlier in my life, I might have tried to insist they come with us, but when I heard his answer, which my husband translated from French, I knew he needed me to do more than **hear** him, he needed me to **listen** to him.

I don't know where or how Daniel's family slept that night or how they did what they did. But Daniel arrived at our house the next morning at 6:30 AM, as he always had, cleaned his mud-covered body and clothes in our compound and brought tea to us in a pristine white cook's uniform at 7:00 AM. He had used his will to make the decisions he made, and was on the job, ready to go, despite adversities incomprehensible to me.

I listened, I watched, and I learned.

A few days later, I stood ankle-deep in mud, in a queue at the Air France desk at Ouagadougou airport. The airport has a dirt floor, like many airports in the global south, and the monsoon season had not yet ended—the rains had not stopped for weeks.

I was flying to Marseille then on to Nice, because I'd decided that I couldn't survive in Burkina Faso unless I learned French, a language I have never studied. This decision came only a few months after we were drop-kicked into living in Burkina Faso, courtesy of the Dutch Development Agency which had posted my husband there. I'd become utterly incapacitated, and frustrated by not knowing a word of French. My work life stopped and when my son became ill with typhoid and malaria, I couldn't speak to health care workers about him. I couldn't even communicate with the household staff. We employed as many as we could to give them an income. Though I had previously spent a decade as CEO of an international organisation working globally, I was now gagged in every aspect of my life. This isolated, landlocked country in West Africa is not like most places I'd visited on that continent, where more than a few people spoke English. Very few Burkinabe spoke anything except for French and Arabic.

I landed at the airport in Nice, France, late at night and thought how surprising it was that I'd spent 20 years running around all the corners of the world but had never visited the South of France. Of course, I'd heard all about the glamourous lifestyle and ritzy villas when I lived in England and travelled around Europe, but I'd written it off as too showy and of no interest for me, so I never visited.

So, why now? A "fixer" by nature, I needed to fix my language problem and had confidently decided—stupidly decided, in retrospect—that I would conquer French in a one-month immersive language school. My research located the best French language immersion program in the world, so I said goodbye to my husband and son at the muddy Ouagadougou airport to spend a month at the *Institut de Francais* in Villefranche-Sur-Mer, on the Mediterranean coast, near Nice. Having landed in Nice late that night, mud-caked jeans still on, I took a cab through the dark to the tiny apartment on a hill that would be my home for the month: French immersion 8:00 AM to 6:00 PM every day, French homework every night.

I quickly learned to love one thing about living in France—*volets*, which are roll-up solid metal shutters that close completely, making interior spaces pitch black, quiet, and entirely secure. Very sensitive to light, I never slept better than in France, thanks to the light-tight *volets*. They were closed when I arrived, so I stumbled into bed, set the alarm early for the classes that were to start the next day, and slept.

Early the next morning, I pushed the button to open the *volets* to the dawn, and my mouth actually dropped open in awe. I'd travelled all over the world but had never seen a more magnificent view than the Bay of Villefranche-Sur-Mer from this lush hillside. I stared at the rugged Mediterranean coastline winding around the Peninsula of Cap Ferrat, with boats gently bobbing in the azure bay. Starting with an expletive, I blurted out, "Why don't I live here?" It truly felt like paradise to me.

A year later, it was our paradise. During that year, my son's health continued to deteriorate in Burkina Faso, so we were transferred, all expenses paid, to any European destination we chose. We chose a village in the South of France, with an English school for my son. So, I found myself sitting in my paradise, on my own balcony, overlooking the Bay of Villefranche-Sur-Mer, where I now lived contentedly with my husband and son. I'd gone from one extreme of life on Earth to the opposite.

Naturally, we found a few snakes in this Eden-like setting. One set of problems was exchanged for another. Burkina Faso was and remains one of the poorest countries on the planet—dirt roads and open sewers, teaming with destitute souls trying to eke out a wage to stay alive every day. Then, almost the next moment, we were on the French Riviera, where there is too much glitz, too much money, and too much excess. But its rugged hillsides, covered with a mix of palms, conifers, and deciduous trees, and bordered by sandy coves and azure bays with yachts happily bobbing, are all shocking beautiful.

When we left Ouagadougou, we gave Daniel a small bonus equivalent to US$50.00—not much to us, but a month's salary for him. A month later, through a friend that had internet, Daniel sent me a picture with a thank you message. He used that money to build a brick wall. He still lived in a mud hut, but one now equipped with a strong barrier defending against the rains that would come the next year. The picture was carefully posed with his large family around him in front of the wall—three wives (he was Muslim), children and grandchildren, all smiling. They listened to Daniel, really heard him and refused to abandon their home. Now, they couldn't believe their luck in getting that wall, and I couldn't believe mine. I was learning to listen, to watch, and learn.

Your Path to Success

Listening as a leader is, in my view, the greatest cornerstone to success among all that you do in any leadership capacity.

People will say they are good listeners because they are in conversation much of time and people appear to enjoy talking to them. Many people (I won't say most, but others might) are not as good at listening as they think they are. Humans tend to dislike silent pauses in conversations. Therefore, we want to answer as soon as a question is asked or interject as soon as an opening arises. We're constantly thinking about and planning what to say next.

When we do that, we aren't listening with our full attention.

Giving the others in a conversation your full attention is the key to good listening. It is the difference between **talking at** someone and **talking with** someone. It's also a demonstration of courtesy, humility, respect, and so on. People need, as well as deserve, that respect just as much as you do.

People need to be heard. We usually discuss ego as a negative, but it isn't entirely so. If you have a healthy and appropriate level of ego, you also have self-respect, self-confidence, and initiative. If you have an ego too low, you're timid, self-conscious, unwilling to "rock the boat." If you have an ego too big, you're perceived as arrogant and self-absorbed. In truth, few people will want to be around you for long because, while you are constantly talking, they've stopped listening, and certainly won't feel heard.

In some parts of Asia they have a concept, usually translated to English as *face*. Your *face* is generally described as a combination of the respect others have for you, your reputation, your honor, and your standing in your various communities. You've probably heard of *saving face* or *losing face*, meaning (in the most simple terms) you did well or did poorly. You either increased or decreased others' good opinion of you.

Another, less discussed, aspect is *giving face* or *taking face*. Your actions can increase or decrease people's good opinion of others. (In so doing, you also gain, or lose, great *face*!) Listening to your people, talking *with* relatives, friends, co-workers, total strangers, giving them your full attention and treating them with the same respect you want to receive from others, increases your *face* and theirs, especially when done publicly. There are *no* negatives attached to this practice. Everybody wins!

Philosophical or metaphysical considerations aside, most people are worth listening to. I have the view that most people have something of interest to say. They could have opinions that could be valuable counsel for your situation. They could have insights that might be answers to questions you have. They could have experiences and skills that you lack. Their bank of knowledge is different from yours. We've spoken already of mentorship, a formal relationship that may least years. Likewise, an informal, unconscious, unintentional relationship may last for one five-minute conversation. If you and I speak with each other, and you gain value from that conversation, I have mentored you for that moment. And you may have likely done the same for me.

Listening to and speaking with (instead of speaking at) others are so fundamental to good human interaction that we should understand them inherently. They should be habits so deeply ingrained in us that they just happen in every interaction. Sadly, we don't live in that world. Many people have to be trained to listen properly. But the good news is that if one is willing to learn there are miraculous gains to be made in human relationships. Undoubtedly, some of the problems women have achieving success, and believing they deserve it, stem from the lack of respect that their superiors, male and female, give them and by not really listening to them.

Don't Just Hear Me Out

If you really listen to someone, rather than just "hearing her out," you will make deeper connections because you can pick up on people's vulnerabilities and their authenticity. Recall my first story about the DFID: I asked the hiring manager for 15 minutes of his time. If he wanted to **appear** to be a truly fine leader, he could've agreed to the meeting, heard me out and said, "Thank you, I appreciate and respect your boldness. I'll reconsider your application and get back to you." If he hadn't really been listening, he'd still have been focused on my negatives and followed up that meeting with another polite rejection.

Instead, he gave me my 15 minutes and **listened** to **me**. That led to a 2-hour conversation because he saw something in me. He didn't focus on my disqualifiers, he focused on a skill set that had potential, despite my lack of experience in his specialized area. He dug deeper and decided that my positives outweighed my negatives, that I had the core of what he wanted and he could train me to do the rest, so he gave me the job then and there. Obviously, that doesn't happen all the time, but isn't it easier to accept a setback when you know the other party fully understood the situation?

It actually goes both ways. I thought the DFID job was just what I needed at that time, but the interviewer knew quite a bit that I didn't. During our dialogue, he could've discovered something about me that would've prevented me from any chance of success in the job, and he could've spared me a failure.

Had the DFID interviewer explained, "This is what we need, you don't have the skills and we don't have the time or budget to train you," or something of that sort, my disappointment would still have been there, but knowing success was impossible would've made the rejection much easier to take.

By listening, you can also pick up on things suggesting a person is qualified but worried that they're not going to make the grade—again, imposter syndrome. You can then judge whether or not those fears are so great that they'll become a self-fulfilling prophecy. To make the right judgment in that situation, you need the connection that only comes from subordinating your desire to control a conversation and by making the other party an equal partner in the dialogue.

In the digital age, driven to unexpected heights by the pandemic, the means and various ways to communicate exploded. Texting and messaging apps have a valuable place in business and everywhere else in society, but they will never replace authentic interpersonal communication.

If I simply need data, phone-to-phone texts along the lines of, "Did you mail that report?" "It went out with yesterday's mail," is perfect.

If you need someone to consider options before replying, an email that starts with, "Here's my idea for a project outline, does it fit your needs?" offers them time to deliberate.

If an immediate response is undesirable, such as when you know the other person is occupied, the message, "I'm ready to go, let me know when you are," not only does the job, it's an expression of courtesy.

Likewise, it's easy to get people together when they all work in the same office. When you need to conference with people in different cities, phone calls have been used for decades, and they still happen. Today, however, we have the added bonus of face-to-face video meetings and screen-sharing tech to literally get everybody on the same page.

The danger lies in getting too comfortable with words or low-resolution images on the screen instead of live communication with a live person. Listening isn't just about hearing words, it's posture, facial expressions, eye contact and other aspects of body language. When practical, a face-to-face real conversation is the best way to get to know the people you work with and live with. Highly emotional intelligent people know there is a lot going on in a room that is beyond the spoken word.

THREE LEVELS OF LISTENING

Co-Active Coaching explains the three levels of listening[7]:

Level 1
Level 1 listening is an interaction where the primary focus of the listener is on their own thoughts, opinions, judgments and feelings. People relate the words they hear to their experiences or needs. This type of listening is entirely appropriate when we are facing a decision or when we must collect information. If we are buying a car, for example, we will be listening at Level 1 to the salesperson to see how the car features will fit our needs and budget. In Level 1 listening, the topic is not high stakes.

---

[7] Laura Whitworth, Henry Kinsey-House & Phil Sandahl, *Co-Active Coaching: New Skills for Coaching People Toward Success in Work and Life* [1st Edition]. Mountain View, CA: Davies-Black Publishing, 1998, accessed 20 June 2022.

Level 2

Level 2 listening takes the communication way ahead. The undivided attention of the listener is entirely on the speaker and on the conversation. This means not only hearing what is being said but also noticing how it is said. It involves paying attention to the tone of voice, body language, and facial expressions. This type is empathic listening, and includes paraphrasing and reflecting on the words of the speaker.

The listener can filter out their internal chatter and any distraction from the environment. As a result, the listener can tune in to the meaning of the words, choose a way to respond, and assess the effect of the response on the speaker. Level 2 listening is a skill that professional coaches use in their communication.

Level 3

Level 3 listening brings an entirely new state of awareness to the conversation. It involves doing everything at Level 2, plus using intuition and being open to receiving more information in any form that it presents itself. This means tuning in not only to the conversation but to the environment.

The use of intuition can be misunderstood because it is not based on hard facts. The concept of intuition is, in fact, simple and can be an excellent communication asset. If you get a hunch, for example, while listening to your conversational partner, consider bringing it up but do not be attached to it. Without insisting on being right, observe the effect it has on the speaker and be aware of where the conversation goes next. It is irrelevant if you are right or wrong; what is important is the effect on the conversation.

CULTIVATE THE ART

LEVEL 1 LISTENING

This is fine for most small topics, housekeeping details, or easy-going water cooler conversations that don't include essential topics.

Level 1 listening, however, turns off certain brain functions in the person listening, possibly giving the speaker the impression that the listener is not interested, not listening, or just self-absorbed. All of these are not leadership traits of leaders who last.

LEVEL 2 LISTENING

A hybrid between Levels 1 and 3, Level 2 is significantly more engaged listening than Level 1. At Level 2, you listen and talk, ask questions and make comments with your own thoughts and perspectives, and the focus may vary between you and the other person. This is fine for topics that have moderate value and when dialogue is needed to resolve a problem.

LEVEL 3 LISTENING

We can all morph between the three levels at all times, but when a crucial topic is on the table, we can and should harness the power to move straight to Level 3 listening. We don't necessarily progress from Level 1 to Level 3 in a conversation, we choose the level appropriate to the time and circumstances. Those circumstances sometimes require us to make a jump from the casual conversation we expected to as serious as it gets, and to make that switch in an instant.

For example, not long ago, my son, Harrison, who lives not far from me in London, called me. His French girlfriend and our family had become very close. We were close to her mother as well. When he called me, he started with, "I've got something to tell you." That could be almost anything, so I, as we tend to do, was listening at Level 1. His girlfriend's mother was young, fit, and healthy, so it was a double shock to hear him say, "She just found that she's riddled with cancer."

In these (thankfully rare) cases, Level 3 hits like a volcanic eruption. Nothing of this was going to be about me. He called me because he was in pain, and they all would need my support. Harrison's father had died of a brain tumor, so I said to him, "This is going to make you relive all that. So you need to try and be prepared for the effect on you while you support her."

Now, suppose that I'd stayed at Level 1 listening. My son calls me and I say, "Hey, hi, how are you? What's going on?" just as we always do. He says, "I've got really bad news, my girlfriend's mother is really ill with cancer." If I respond, "Oh, yeah, I had a friend with that kind of cancer once. I hope she'll be okay."

This is why I use that word, **highjack** with respect to conversations. In this scenario, Level 1 listening wouldn't put the focus on the priority issues—a woman possibly facing a death sentence, her daughter who loves her, and my son's ability to manage that situation, which is and will be difficult for some time. Level 1 listening would have made it about me, my experience. I wouldn't have given him the respect he needed to stay with his own sadness, through listening support. He didn't ask me for help. He only needed me to deeply listen.

I generally don't give anybody advice unless they ask for it, even my children. But in that case, I'd seen how devastated my kids were when their dad was taken, and I wanted him to be ready. Fortunately, he was, "Yeah, I'm already feeling like it's *deja vu* for me." So I said, "But you'll be a great support for her because you've lived through this." And, he was and still is. (And she's doing great now!)

It's a question of severity. Level 1 is casual. Level 2 is important. Level 3 is crucial. You never know where a conversation will go, so you have to be flexible. That requires paying attention because the speaker may not come out and explode their troubles to your face. Many times, people want you, the listener, to take the initiative and say, "What's wrong? Are you OK?" They are, in effect, seeking your permission to up the exchange to Level 3. If you're not paying attention to tone, cadence, and other clues, you risk them leaving the conversation without the help you might've given, the help they needed.

On top of all that, you need to be brave. Sometimes, it is the courage to be quiet. At other times, it is the courage to speak the truth people don't want to hear. We need to be direct but in compassionate ways. The truth can be brutal, but there's never a reason to be brutal to other people.

LEVEL 0 — NOT LISTENING

There really isn't a level 0, but there are bad habits we can easily fall into which can end effective listening and some that aren't bad ideas in themselves, they just don't fit the particular situation.

Principally, listening problems stem from that heightened ego I mentioned earlier. Many of us naturally want to be seen as smart, to be seen as fixing problems, and some have the bad habit of needing to have the last word. Being smart, fixing a problem, putting a final thought on a subject are fine. But if you feel the need to do it with every conversation, ask yourself, "Why?" Did it really help the other party or was it just so you looked good to yourself or others? Some people's egos are stroked when they push people around, they bully them into following their advice, or just so they can have their "badge" of brutality, say what they think as harshly as possible, then move on and to hell with people's feelings.

Of course, there are people who don't really care, they just love to hear themselves talk. Go to them and ask for advice and the dialogue is over. You'll never get another word in, as they drone on and on.

None of that is fun and none is helpful. And this book definitely isn't for those types of people.

Similarly, there are some who may come to you for advice, but don't really want to listen to you. They reject every idea with a very negative attitude that suggests to you they don't really want advice or aren't willing to do what it takes to solve their problem or whatever. If you're being ignored, you tend to tune down to Level 1 listening at that point, because, they aren't actually listening to you. Remember that your own time has more value, and end the conversation.

PRACTICAL FACTORS

Test Yourself on these habits of **Level 1** Listening:

1. Are you high-jacking someone's point to focus the attention on you?
2. Are you changing the subject with little or no segue?
3. Are you asking questions, but not paying attention to the answers?

Test Yourself on these habits of **Level 3** Listening:

1. Are you both physically and mentally quiet when others speak?
2. Are you asking questions about what the speaker has said without bringing focus back to yourself?

3. Are you making eye contact?
4. Are you refraining from fiddling with things, phones, keys, acting distracted?
5. Have you asked if they are able to look at it any other ways, with other viewpoints?
6. Have you asked what they need from you on this topic? Is it just to listen? To give ideas? To suggest actions?
7. Are you prepared to do absolutely nothing, except listen, because the other isn't ready for advice, they just need to know you care?

Level 2 is the in-between, mixing the aspects of **Level 1** and **Level 3**. It's where most of us naturally find ourselves. **Level 3** listening is a habit to be cultivated, where you remember that moments of silence matter. You simply need to consciously decide that you'll pay attention, and value, what others have to say. Perhaps most difficult of all, to understand what they need.

CHAPTER 6

NICE & KIND DON'T MEAN WEAK

The waiting is the hardest part
Every day you see one more card
You take it on faith, you take it to the heart
The waiting is the hardest part.

—Tom Petty, "The Waiting"

INTRODUCTION — FOUR-LETTER WORDS – NICE, KIND, WEAK

Do you think you are kind, nice, weak, aggressive, assertive, brassy, feisty (a word I despise, does anyone ever call a man "feisty"?), warm, authentic, energetic, charming, compelling, or off-putting? Have you ever been told you are any of these? I think someone has thought of me in every one of those terms at one time or another. Some of those views might have some merit but most are labels put on me by people who know too little about me to have a valid opinion.

Or have you been told, as I was by a male colleague, that you should not smile and laugh so much, or you would not be considered a "professional" executive? In today's world, few people might not say such a thing to your face because our politically-correct world would pounce on them, but many people still think this way.

It's a confusing time we live in, with the terms like "gender equality" and "gender equity" thrown around haphazardly, meaning different things to different people, leaving some of us confused. Some men still want to rely on old-fashioned manners and protocols while others say to women, "You wanted equality, so you got it. I'm not opening a door for you."

It's a baffling world and many people are justifiably confused with who they are and how they should act and be perceived and how they could act so that they feel and appear confident and assertive, without the labels that get thrown onto our actions.

You can be assertive without being aggressive. How? Calibrate your tone, be **firm**, not **shrill** and speak in a low-toned, conversational manner. Earn a reputation for being **calm** and **kind**, but **clear** and **concise**. Hold your head straight and watch the body language of your role models. See how many women (but very few men) tilt their head to the side when they're hesitant about what they're saying. You can be firm and empathetic because they are not opposites. They can be complementary. You can be kind without being weak. Most importantly, **think before you speak and act**. You can do this in a nanosecond if you train your mind. After years of considering how to calibrate and prepare what I say, it's now second nature. But I'm still **practicing** that skill, and I always will.

I try to deliver information in a way that's beneficial, rather than detrimental, when stakes are high and conversations have high risks but potentially high returns. I learned a method from the former mediator and relationship expert, Paul Friedman, called SEW, which he outlined in his fascinating book *Breaking The Cycle*.[8] Paul's acronym stands for, "Stop, Evaluate, and act with Wisdom."

I have my own version I call SEAP, **"Stop, Evaluate and Act with care after Practice."** I apply this to my personal and professional life when I know or just sense there's a crucial conversation about to happen. I rehearse many crucial conversations in my head before they happen, so I'm as prepared as possible for whatever turn the conversation may take. (More on this in the next chapter.) Through regular practice, I have reserves in my toolbox for many possible bumps in the conversational road.

Making a habit of practicing what you'll say in various scenarios gives you *power*—it preserves your free will. You've heard people say something like, "I got so angry I just couldn't help myself!" That's a real problem—anybody can get so angry that common sense and self-control go out the window. When you speak in anger or because of some other stress, you are *reactive, not responsive*. You lose control when you act based on external stimuli. When you speak, having practiced and prepared, you are *proactive*

[8] Paul Friedman, *Breaking The Cycle, Updated Edition*. San Marcos, CA: The Marriage Foundation, 2012, accessed 21 June 2022.

and responsive. You maintain control of your emotions and, therefore, your free will.

Many women I meet and speak with think that expressing vehement anger or letting a temper show makes them appear strong. While I feel anger at many of the injustices of the world, I think women lose power when they cannot keep their anger under control.

Some of the most powerful people in the world show feeling, speak firmly, but innately know that showing aggression with anger openly means weakness. Think of Angela Merkel, the former Chancellor of Germany, considered one of the strongest female leaders of this generation. Did you ever see her angry? No. Did you see her be firm? Yes. Michelle Obama? The same. I'm not saying you shouldn't have strong feelings, nor that you should never get angry about situations that are unjust. We have feelings and the right to own those feelings, but as Paul Friedman says, you also have choice—free will—to choose how you respond to provoking behaviours or actions, labelling by others, or other bad manners. You don't have to be controlled by what others do. Control yourself, and exhibit anger with control.

Have you ever been told you are "too aggressive" for a woman? Have you been called "ballsy"? The reference to male anatomy, when applied to a woman, is always negative and entirely inappropriate. However, references to a man as "ballsy" is considered positive, he's being "assertive," right? (Maybe, but references to genitalia are still absolutely inappropriate in business settings.) Despite that, he gets accolades for being "strong" and "outspoken"—both compliments—but, when a woman does it, she is called "aggressive" and "feisty"—both criticisms.

When I hear these things, I do get angry, and I assume you do as well, but I control my response to it. Many very accomplished women I speak with have told me they have trouble associating "assertiveness" with "angry" because, when a woman is called assertive, it usually means people perceive her as overly-aggressive and that simply isn't true. Women want to be seen as assertive, but "assertive" is neither "arrogant" nor "aggressive." It is firm, solid, and emotionally intelligent. It simply means you are willing to move forward without waiting for an invitation or being told to go ahead.

THE STUDENTS

A few years ago, I was teaching a course in behavioural economics to MBA students at *Ipag Ecole Supérieure de Commerce* in Nice, one of France's top business schools. At the beginning of the term, I always told my class of very professionally-accomplished students, "Come to class, do the reading, do the writing, engage with me and the others, speak your mind, listen carefully, and you'll do well."

But, every term, there is a person (sometimes two) who simply doesn't prep for classes. I know who they are by our third session. They don't join in class discussions because they clearly have not done the reading prep. Every term, I ask those one or two students to stay after class for a chat. If there are two, I see them together.

I ask them if they are enjoying the business school, if they're enjoying Nice, what about France, and, lastly, I ask if they enjoy my class. When (not if) they say, "Yes, of course," I ask them, "How do you know? Because you've missed class and you're not engaging with me or other students because you can't. You clearly haven't read the prep materials."

Then I wait. Like Tom Petty sang, "Waiting is the hardest part."

There are usually a few excuses about being busy, and other nonsense, however, soon enough, they're saying something like, "But you seemed so *nice* that first week. Why are you hassling us now?" or "You seemed so *kind* that first class, saying you would try to be tolerant of issues and problems and offer help where possible!" or "Well, I got busy," they tell, me, "no big deal to miss a class or some reading."

I wait a few seconds after they're finished, so I can think through my response. Then I smile a bit and, speaking in a low tone, I tell them, "One of the best lessons you will ever learn in business is that **nice** and **kind** do not mean **weak**. If you start with those preconceived notions about a person, you will fail every time. And you'll fail this course, which you need to pass to get your MBA, a degree that some sponsor or benevolent person who believes in you, paid handsome fees for you to be here to achieve. You make your choice."

And then I wait again. I am offering them an opportunity to exercise their free will.

And guess what? Those one or two students are the ones who turn into the model students and almost always end up doing well in the course.

ATTITUDES & ACTIONS

Can I define **nice**, **kind**, and **weak**?

To me, a **nice** person has an attitude—one who is not aggressive, but inclusive. She's agreeable and non-contentious, but it's a more unstructured term. "She was really nice," often simply means, "She was really friendly"—courteous and smiling, for example. I'm one of those who smiles often though I've met people who never have any soft facial expressions.

The French commonly say, "Don't smile so much." The British, at least in previous generations, had a reputation for "keeping the stiff upper lip"—a tradition of unemotional stoicism in public life, which often carried over to private life. Americans, many studies show, tend to smile too much, in the opinions of foreigners. Personally, I prefer to err on the side of a pleasant expression and good attitude.

When teaching that MBA course, I tried to be nice, kind, and understanding. That is my nature. I tried to sincerely be a little extra nice to those students because they were nervous—all different cultures, in a new city, some already very incredibly accomplished but unsure of themselves. "I only speak five languages, Jill, can I get a good job?" I was asked more than once. A lot of them had 10 years of career experience behind them, so I knew they were capable, but I tried to be nice just to draw us together as a group, so they'd achieve greater success.

I kept my approach as simple as possible:

- Look them in the eye.
- Ask them where they're from.
- Ask them what they want to get out of the course.
- Ask them if they have any worries about the process they're going to go through.
- Ask them what they hoped to do with their degree.

I was simply interested in them as people. I did, naturally, have a vested interest in helping them achieve success in my course, but I am authentically interested in almost every person I come across. It doesn't always work out, of course. There are people I meet and come away thinking, "Yeah, once is quite enough." But I can find something interesting in almost everybody I meet, whether it's the builder fixing the back door or a senior politician or executive. There's an old proverb, "If you're interested, you're interesting." Lucky for me, I'm interested in many subjects. I look for those things in others. I've always subscribed to the idea that you should seek out some way to connect positively with everyone you meet.

Likewise, a **kind** person is one whose actions show empathy. When you perceive that a problem exists, either because someone asks for help or you simply see a potential need, you think, "I'm going to look and listen; really understand what's going on from their perspective. I'm going to create a safe space for them to share what they need to share, so they feel that there is someone who cares about the outcome of their situation. Then (and only then) I act to create a positive outcome—one that meets their **true needs**, not simple the need I might see from my perspective.

Kindness has a very magnetic form of charm. There's so much negativity, so much aggression, so much of every bad attitude in the world today, if you project an air of kindness, people are naturally drawn to you. When they believe that you'll do something for them "just because," you'll find them more ready to do something for you "just because."

I'm not suggesting round after round of *quid pro quo*—doing favors so people will owe you favors. When you are kind to others and people understand that you're doing it with no expectation of ever having that kindness repaid, most of them will adopt that same attitude toward you. They may even be inspired to "pay it forward" to others in need.

We all prefer to be around nice, kind people, and being a nice, kind person is the fastest way to attract them. I firmly believe, and no one has ever given me a reason to think otherwise, that all humans deserve this—that these traits are the lubrication that makes the machine that is human society work well and right.

But sometimes, tough people see those with this attitude as **weak** people. I've never seen it that way. I see weak people as those who have no impulse control, those who change their minds each time someone says "I don't want to do that." They're over-acquiescent, without the confidence to stand their ground when they have a position that they don't think should change. Or, they're so tough because inside they are racked with insecurity and toughness is their wall to protect them. If you move your position because of other people's pressure on you, I'd say you're giving in to weakness.

This may link into imposter syndrome—if you don't think you should be in charge, you'll subconsciously hand over control to others.

This may also link into a need (conscious or subconscious) to be liked, without the self-confidence to be liked for what you are instead of what you can do for someone else. Too many women believe, "If I agree with them, they'll like me. If I don't agree, they won't like me." To a point, that may be true, but that is their problem, not yours. I once heard an old US Navy maxim, "The first rule of command is to command." For our purposes, let me combine and rephrase those two ideas:

"When you're hired to make the right decision, make that right decision. If others dislike that decision, or you for making it, that's on them. You cannot live your life trying to live up to others' expectations."

Sure, it would be great if everyone liked me, but I don't expect it. I'm not everybody else's cup of tea and they aren't mine. I'm not going to change what I believe in just to get somebody to like me, and I will never recommend that anyone do that. Be kind, be nice, but, above all, be genuinely your authentic self.

BENEFITS TO THE WORKPLACE

Co-workers are a team, and you'll be on one team or another for your entire working life. You want to connect to teammates because it makes the workflow and the workplace better. Philosophically, people want to be part of something bigger than themselves. Practically, team successes translate to individual successes and those translate to promotions, pay increases, better offers, and personal job satisfaction.

The 21st Century has brought situations that strain the whole idea of unity and cooperation. There is global aggression and the idea that my neighbor may be my enemy in disguise. We've experienced a pandemic and the related medical, societal, operational and political issues. There are other challenges too numerous to name. We need, like few of us have ever needed in our lifetimes, nicer behaviour and kinder action. We need to value our teammates (and other people in general) more because there are forces in the world dedicated to breaking down people's unity, self-esteem, and general success. Connections, professional and personal, build self-esteem and success in others and that building, by its nature, expands your own self-esteem and success.

Nice is the attitude that inspires kind acts and those are the building blocks of team spirit. They are two of the cornerstones of team success.

Benefits to the Community

Whenever I'm kind to somebody—give them some of my time, give them some of my thoughts, give any type of help when I see them struggling—I've felt better about myself. I'm glad that I took the time to do something that didn't profit me in any material way. I just made someone else's life better, because I could.

Like any parent, I've had to deal with my children going through rough days. I've always counseled them, "When you're having a tough time, feeling anxious or worried, or whatever, find something to look forward to, even if it's a cup of tea, or a holiday or, better still, do something for somebody else." You don't have to focus on anything new or even anything big. Just find something to look forward to so you can put your brain in that moment instead of the present, less-than-happy moment. Even better, go do something for somebody else. Go volunteer somewhere; make a donation to a charity, take your neighbor a cake. That has always worked for me. When life challenges you, connect to someone else. It relieves stress and anxiety.

My daughter, Hannah, now a successful professional woman living in New York, has been struggling with a chronic health issue, which she has managed since she was diagnosed at 12 years old, despite the chronic pain that accompanies it. During the pandemic, at Christmas season, she adopted an old cat from the shelter. She said, "I'm going to take an old one and I'm going to love it to death"—quite literally—"I'm going to do something nice for that cat that nobody wants because it is not a kitten, and I'm going to do something nice for myself by loving it." Those are the moments that make a mother proud.

I want to emphasise that little things can be just as important as major acts. Some people can make a large donation to charity, which is great, but most charities would be equally grateful for a small donation, because small donations add up. More importantly, any donation or act of kindness also makes you feel better about yourself.

Benefits to You

Be kind to yourself. If you can't do that, it's not likely you'll do well being kind to others.

Check In or Check Out, as Needed

To me, it's always about balance. My partner came into my office one day and asked what I was doing.

"I'm preparing for a meeting with my publisher. I need to get some things straight in my head for that meeting, which is coming up soon. I've been doing things for everybody else all day, and now I need to look at my own stuff, to put me first for a while."

That day, I had a girlfriend with a personal problem and I spent an hour on the phone with her. My daughter called with a professional problem and I spent an hour on the phone with her. I had all these items on my headhunting To-Do list, because that's my job. We had some new work come in, which is great. I could've worked late into the night on that stuff but, then I thought, "No, I'm going to take *me* out at six o'clock. I'm going to take me and nobody else is getting me."

Checking in with yourself so you can balance all the roles you have to play is an important part of giving to others. I believe in giving, but I don't believe in giving only to others because, if you don't give to yourself, you'll run out of reserves. You shouldn't feel bad about giving to yourself; the more you give to yourself, the more you have to give to others. So, when needed, check out of all your other responsibilities and check in with yourself.

BE SELF-AWARE NOT SELF-ABSORBED

Ayn Rand, famed as the author of novels like *Atlas Shrugged* and *The Fountainhead* (both written decades ago, but relevant today) also wrote several essays on this topic:

> In popular usage, the word *selfishness* is a synonym of evil; the image it conjures is of a murderous brute who tramples over piles of corpses to achieve his own ends ... and pursues nothing but the gratification of the mindless whims of any immediate moment.
>
> Yet the exact meaning and dictionary definition of the word *selfishness* is: concern with one's own interests.
>
> This concept does not include a moral evaluation; it does not tell us whether concern with one's own interests is good or evil; nor does it tell us

what constitutes man's [or woman's] actual interests. It is the task of ethics to answer such questions.[9]

Rand and many other authors have followed her lead in this vital issue of keeping yourself mentally and emotionally healthy so that you have strength to share with others. Perhaps "self-aware" is a better term for the 21st Century mentality. What you call it isn't so important as the idea: Maintain the balance of giving in your life to keep your reserves full.

ACCEPT INEVITABLE DEFEATS

There's a professional man I have been keeping my eye on in my headhunting job. We've known each other for a long time now. He's a very capable senior vice president in a bank who needed a change of job and I've put him up for five different jobs. For all five, he's come in number two. Each time the bad news arrived, he just said, "That's the way it went. Let's try again." Each time he thanked me sincerely for putting him forward. Finally, just before this book went to press, he came in number one—on his sixth try—and I was jumping for joy! He handled each rejection with grace and good nature. He was kind, nice, but never weak.

Every day, I talk to people about jobs. I generally forward the top six candidates to the hiring organization, meaning five disappointments on every search. Some take the bad news stoically, like this man did, others

---

[9] Ayn Rand & Nathaniel Branden, *The Virtue of Selfishness: A New Concept of Egoism.* New York City: Signet Books, 1964.

are crushed emotionally. They have put heart and soul into getting the job. They envision themselves in the job, often in a new location which involves an international move; new schools if they have children; new cultures; a secondary language becoming their primary; the list goes on. Handing out the bad news is the worst part of my job and, in every search, it happens five times as often as I get to send out good news. When the magic doesn't happen, that's when women really need to be brave, stoic, and resilient. When you get stuck in a tricky spot, the worst thing you can do is stop!

Second Chances, Seeing the Potential in others

I wrote earlier of my "juvenile delinquent" days. My daughter, Hannah, was always pretty easy to handle. We had to deal with her illness, which was difficult, but as a person, she was never argumentative or problematic. My son, Harrison, was the apple that didn't fall far from the maternal half of the family tree. I actually called the police on him when he was 14. It was tough empathy to be sure. When they came to the door, I took them into the kitchen:

"My son's doing drugs, I've just discovered there is pot and hash all over my house."

They asked, "Where is he?" Then this big, burly cop said, "Leave me alone with him."

"Okay," I said, not knowing where that agreement would take us all. With our home's open floor plan, I hear some of what was going on in the other room, but not much. I did clearly hear Harrison giving the officer a lot of backtalk, saying things like, "Oh, you're on private property. You can't do anything to me."

The officer came in the kitchen and said, "Madam, have I your agreement to arrest your son?"

I said, "Yes, you can." So, they handcuffed my son and took him to jail. Several hours later, about 4:00 AM, to be precise, I got a phone call which startled me awake out of bad sleep. When your 14-year old son is in jail you don't sleep so well!

The officer on the line said to me, "M'am, your son is 14 years old. I don't want him to have a record. He's a smartass, but he's got his whole life ahead of him. If you want to come and get him, you can. No record this time, but if it happens again, he's going to get a criminal record."

I sighed a long sigh of relief, but the problem wasn't solved yet. His attitude had not improved substantially in his time as a would-be jailbird. That was about the time we were called on to relocate to Burkina Faso. Then came his illnesses—typhoid and malaria—followed by our time in France, where his headmaster said to me: "He shouldn't even be here as a high school student. He's lived around the world. He's lived in West Africa. He's gone through trauma, and he's too old, mentally, to be here, even though he's just 17. His dad is dying of a brain tumour. He needs to get out there and be in the world." Harrison had bad grades but at the International School in Ougadougou he won the Barack Obama award for high potential.

We were then living in France and Harrison hoped to go to University in the UK where he'd grown up. So, he applied to ask five universities for a place. His grades were non-existent and four universities wrote back saying, in essence, "You've got to be joking."

That hit him the way Stockbridge (my boarding school experience) hit me. After the fourth refusal, he sat for a while, just muttering, "I'm going to be pumping gas all my life or I'm going to be asking, 'Do you want fries with that?'" (Always witty is Harrison, even in light of a bad situation.)

The light went on for him, as it had for me. And then, a miracle happened. The fifth school, Kingston University in London called to invite him for an interview. What? How did he get an interview? But his Dad and I took him to that interview, and when we arrived, the Head of the Geography Dept. At Kingston said:

"Could I have Harrison on his own for a few hours?" We left him, bewildered and waiting.

After that interview, he got an unconditional offer from the school! In the UK, it's common to get conditional offers of enrollment in university based on final grades, meaning you only get to attend if your final grades are very, very good. The only subject Harrison had shown any interest in was geography, and that was only enough to earn a C, while failing everything else in high school. Why did Harrison get an unconditional offer to attend Kingston?

A lot of the parents at his high school were seriously unhappy when news of this got around. Some asked, "What strings did you pull?" I hadn't pulled any. I think the people at Kingston saw some potential in him. They said, in effect, "This is a person with tons of potential, but he hasn't realized it yet." I also secretly thought, at that time (and I still do), that the kind headmaster of his French high school called Kingston and told them Harrison might not have the grades, but definitely had the intellect and potential.

At university, Harrison soared. He got merits—he graduated with honors—from Kingston, followed by offers from all the best Masters programmes in the United Kingdom. He went to the University of Lancaster, again graduating with honors in Energy and Environment. Now, he has a professional executive job, working in energy, and is becoming hugely successful. About a year ago in fact, as I was writing this book, I got in touch with Professor Garside, his department head at Kingston (who still teaches there), who gave him the unconditional offer. The Professor combined much of what we've been discussing on kindness and putting faith in someone's potential, and he made a huge difference for my son. In fact, when I contacted him to thank him for seeing the potential in Harrison, he asked if Harrison would come and speak to the students about how life can turn out when you see the potential in someone. Harrison did, of course, with great success.

During all this, I've often thought, "Oh, now I know how my mom felt," and I told Mom many times, "I'm so sorry for being so problematic." My mother was, right up until she passed away, a very forgiving, non-judgmental person. She'd always reply with something like, "Well, that's what happened, and you make me really proud now." I've now had that same conversation with my own son, who makes be proud every day.

We all need a second chance at some point and we all need to give them to others. Try your best to see the potential in yourself and in others.

Build a Legacy

Courtesy and kindness, accepting defeat graciously instead of angrily, giving ourselves and others second chances, avoiding the weakness of acquiescence— these, of course, are short-term thinking as we interact with others on a day-to-day basis. There is also long-term thinking to do: The notion of **legacy**.

You might be surprised I'm writing so much about your relationship with yourself. You shouldn't be. "Charity begins at home," they say, and you must be good at being kind to yourself before you can be really good at being kind to others. I started this chapter by saying "a **nice** person is an attitude. It is one who is not aggressive, but inclusive." Would you ever consider excluding yourself? Some people actually do, but normally no, we like ourselves better than we like anybody else. And that's where it needs to start. Our self-image is the cornerstone of everything in our lives, all that we might accomplish. And those accomplishments form our legacy.

I've always been interested in mortality because I'm not a person of faith but of spirituality. I maintain a view somewhere between atheist and agnostic. I like to feel that there's some sort of spirit that goes on after we leave Earth, but I stay focused in this life because that's what I'm sure of. I think we're here for however long we're here, and what happens afterwards, if anything, is outside my understanding. So, a personal legacy becomes that much more important. I like the adage attributed to Stephen Grellet:

> I expect to pass through this world but once. Any good, therefore, that I can do or any kindness I can show to any fellow creature, let me do it now. Let me not defer or neglect it, for I shall not pass this way again.[10]

It's important that we remind ourselves of our own mortality, so we are encouraged to live a good life while we can. Successful people have learned not to procrastinate in their activities. Don't procrastinate building your legacy. Many people question, "What will my legacy be?" while others wonder, "Will I have a legacy?" The short answer is, "Everyone will have a

---

[10] Étienne de Grellet du Mabillier, later known simply as "Stephen Grellet" (1772-1855), was a French-American missionary. Born in Limoges, France, to a prominent family, he fled to South America during the French Revolution, eventually arriving in the United States in 1795. Joining the Society of Friends (commonly called "Quakers"), he ministered extensively in prisons and hospitals across North American and Europe. The quote is most commonly attributed to him, and there is some evidence of his authorship, but it is disputed.

legacy. It will be as good or bad, as notable or obscure, as you make it."

What parts of you will live on after you've "shuffled off this mortal coil"?[11] Perhaps some physical or academic creations—the things you've written or painted or built or knowledge you've added to the human corpus. Perhaps friends and co-workers who'll cherish your memory for your coaching, leadership, and mentoring, as well as the profits your labour earned them. Certainly, your *face*, the reputation you earned during your lifetime.

Like anything else, you have a certain control—considerable power, in fact—over your legacy. I would assume the greatest kindness that you can do yourself is to live a life such that you'll leave behind a better world for the rest of us. Then again, if that's too much to contemplate, maybe just one small corner of it that's better. Either way, you'll be remembered fondly, as an example others will strive to emulate.

CONCLUSION

I think the most famous line from *The Godfather* movies is the repeated phrase, "It's nothing personal, it's just business."[12] The fictional Corleone family used that simple sentence to justify the most heinous crimes imaginable. More than anything else, they used it to

---

[11] William Shakespeare, *Hamlet*, Act 3, Scene 1, Line 67.
[12] *The Godfather*, Paramount Pictures, 1972; *The Godfather, Part II*, Paramount Pictures, 1974; *The Godfather, Part III*, Paramount Pictures, 1990.

lie to themselves, to convince themselves they are not the evil people that they truly were.

That, of course, is the most extreme example possible, but we're all capable of that same self-deception. Anyone who truly believes that business is not personal is kidding themselves. Because we're human, everything is, at least, a little bit personal. Business success, in fact, is often based on personal relationships—the trust, respect, and attitudes others develop for or about you. In short, again, your *face*. And, of course, the same that you develop for others. It all goes to credibility and credibility is vital.

It's **never** just business—your co-workers, vendors, contractors, clients, and every other stakeholder is a person. They have needs, goals, fears. Never forget that, to each of them, it will, at some point, be **very** personal.

CHAPTER 7

WINNING HABITS OF BRAVE (AND SUCCESSFUL) WOMEN

There's a special place in hell for women that don't help other women.

— Madeleine Albright, former US Secretary of State, speech celebrating the WNBA's All-Decade Team, 2006

INTRODUCTION — THE GOOD, THE BAD, THE UGLY

[NOT NECESSARILY IN THAT ORDER.]

Early in my career, I was appointed Manager of Public Relations for North America for Hyatt Hotels. I was just 25, so had a few years under my belt, but was looking for female role models. I was hired after several tough interviews, including a few with my potential direct supervisor, a woman in her late thirties. During the extensive interview process, she was open, charming, and supportive.

On my first day in the job, she criticised the business suit I was wearing, swore at me, gave me press releases to draft, and then took her red pen to savage them. Her face the colour of her pen, she would burst into my office, just across from hers, with floor to ceiling glass walls, throwing red-marked documents on my desk, scribbled with expletives. What came out of her mouth in these outbursts was more of the same—loud and angry.

For two years, I continued working in this environment, not knowing when I arrived in the office each day (early every day) whether she would sing-song "Good morning!" or shout "Get the *fuck* in my office, right now!"

She confused solving a problem—my style of writing, which was raw back then but improved over time— with creating stress and controversy. I spent many long nights up with a colleague and friend trying to decide if I should go to HR to complain or go over her head to her boss, or simply quit. I've always believed that going over the head of your boss can be suicide, but after getting a lukewarm response from HR, who simply shrugged and said, "Well, we know about her but that's the way she is." I went to her boss; at that point, I had nothing to lose.

I had come to the place where it was quit or seek advice from her supervisor. So, I asked for a meeting with her boss, the Vice President. He made time for me privately. To my surprise, when I told him the situation and that I was near resigning, he calmly said, "Don't let her do it."

What? How would I just "not let her do it"? He explained that he would intervene if he had to, but that I was fully capable of managing this situation. He told me he had faith in me and that the next time she treated me in an aggressive and disrespectful way, I should simply say, "I'll speak to you about this topic only if we mutually speak in a respectful tone, without angry shouting and aggressiveness." I went home that night, thought hard about whether I could actually do this, and decided to be brave.

The next morning when she shouted, "Jill, get the *fuck* in my office, **now**!" I went into her office, and when she started delivering the loud angry diatribe at me, I was terrified, but said, as the VP advised, "I'll speak to you about this only if we mutually speak in a respectful tone, without angry shouting and aggressiveness." I then turned and walked out of her office and into mine and sat down. Unsurprisingly, she went ballistic and came after me. I repeated the same again and, after the third repetition, she stormed out and left the office. I did not see her again that day.

The next day, and every day afterwards, she never raised her voice, she never wrote the red scribbled expletives, I never saw the shouting red face. I took her (now calm and helpful) suggestions on how to improve very seriously. I learned many lessons there, but perhaps the most valuable lesson is that being motivated by fear never solves problems, it only corrupts and creates tension.

Years later, in my work for SRI Executive, my task is to find the best people on the planet to run UN agencies and other international organisations. It's fascinating and challenging but hugely rewarding work when we get it right, which is most of the time.

As you now know, for each of these roles, I'm assigned a lead research associate who manages the global search through several means, connecting with our staff around the world in sourcing great people.

A highly skilled, fantastically efficient research lead is a dream for a consultant like me working in this field. I think of those coming up after me in one of three categories: The **gold** leads have huge career potential within them. The **silver** leads might get to the top, but it isn't certain to me yet, maybe they simply need more time to let their potential show. The **pewter** people simply don't have what it takes. They have a low EI/ EQ, are sloppy in their work, aren't mission-driven, or are simply wrong for the job. They are the ones that need to find different work if they don't want to sink to the bottom.

Recently, we were challenged to find a very high-level position in the UN and I was assigned Sidney as research lead. Sidney and I had never worked together, and I admit I had some hesitancy about working with a new person for such a crucial role. But Sidney turned out to be double gold. She thought of issues before I did. She practiced tough empathy with the candidates and the client. She handled herself in a warm-yet-professional and highly-organised way. I love a number two who always knows what we need and works with me in full collaboration. But only a **gold** can do this.

Because she showed early on that she was capable, I gave her far more responsibility than I might have given to a **silver** number two. I would've helped a **silver** person learn and grow because that's also part of my job as a female leader and a supervisor. It's also my responsibility as a person. If I had been assigned a **pewter**, I would have asked for somebody else, but there aren't many **pewters** at SRI. Using the wrong people is a risk for the company and the client, especially at our level, and it's never worth it. It would've meant a major loss of reputation for our organization, for SRI Executive, and for me.

Happily, none of that happened. We closed the deal, found the best person for the role and, after months of rigorous interviews and evaluation, including some to measure emotional intelligence, the offer was made and accepted. I sent Sidney a short note, saying how much I valued and appreciated her fantastic help, and I also told the CEO of SRI Executive that she was senior consultant material, even before I had given Sidney that compliment. About the same time, Sidney wrote me a note:

> "Jill, a piece of feedback for you that I want to highlight is that I very much appreciated your support in letting me "step up." I want to progress and move into a consultant role soon, and you provided just the right amount of space and support to enable that. So, thank you!"

Sidney had nailed it and I was grateful to her. We need to give people the balance of support and space to do what they can to build themselves, in skills, self-esteem, and confidence. Shortly after that exchange, Sidney was promoted to Consultant. I was overjoyed for her.

My first supervisor at Hyatt Hotels totally missed the mark in our early years together. She allowed anger to cloud her response to my need for training and mentorship. Through that experience and many others, I developed a personal system that helped me coach and teach up-and-coming women some of the skills they'd need for success.

Looking back, I think the most significant realization that came to me as I was reading, and afterwards, was the idea that there are **simple practices** that you can put in place which can dramatically improve the way you feel and think about your life as a whole. With that as my cue, I have devised these habits of highly successful women:

1. THE "MORE OF/LESS OF" EXERCISE

When I had an in-office staff, before I began working from home, I frequently used the "more of, less of" exercise. I mentioned this in a previous chapter, but it needs more detail here. It's a way to give and receive feedback that's low-key and gentle. I find most people are naturally reluctant to give feedback, particularly feedback that could be construed as negative or critical. Conventional wisdom says see the good things first, and I agree, but this exercise replaces "What am I doing well?" and "What am I doing badly?" with "What do I want to see more of?" and "What do I want to see less of?" It can get exactly the same information but, psychologically, those terms are a lot easier for us to handle.

Start by drawing a line down the middle of a piece of paper (very Old School, here) with "More of" at the top of one side and "Less of" on the other:

- I start with positives then flow gently into the negatives in a courteous, professional fashion.
- It can be done one-on-one (my general preference) but also works in a group setting to evaluate the team as a whole. Once somebody starts contributing, the other team members naturally start contributing.
- Having used it many years, I feel like it takes the sting out of a call to improve, and builds self-esteem by reinforcing what's working.

For example: I might say to an associate, "I really appreciate the fact that you come in and say hello to me every morning when you get a coffee" or "I really value the fact that you always meet your deadlines." Whatever it is, little or big, mention it. I can then transition to suggesting improvements.

This works up the chain as well as down. When a project concludes, my team reviews my performance. They might say, I'd like you to check in with me less often because it makes me feel like you don't trust what I'm doing" or "I'd like you to agree less quickly to what we suggest in afternoon meetings. Go home and think it over, then come in the next morning and share your opinion on the suggestion." (That was a surprise, but they felt strongly about it, so, I did try hard to do that.)

This process makes it very easy for me to see what they appreciate and also what I should be doing to be a better manager and a better leader.

2. VALUE FEEDBACK TO YOURSELF AND OTHERS

Feedback has two components, the process and the result, as an article from the newspaper *Houston Chronicle* describes:

> Performance feedback is a communications process. It should be ongoing, meaning adjustments are made based on the information exchanged between manager and team member. There should be regular follow up dialogue to determine success. ...
>
> Performance feedback is useless unless business leaders have standards for performance, meaning they should have expectations of reasonable achievement. For example, a car dealership may set the standard as 10 sales per month. ... Without these standards, a manager is unable to take a baseline level of productivity and make adjustments.
>
> When it comes to adjustments, leaders need to get the feedback from the team member before they can provide new goals and tasks for improvement. The employee unable to meet 10 car sales per month might be struggling because he is not getting scheduled for the prime sales periods. In most cases, the only way a manager can provide effective feedback is

to be among the team. A sports coach can't provide productive feedback without seeing a player do his job. The feedback from the team member is as important as the feedback the manager provides. In fact, it is how the manager is able to fully understand the situation and make the right adjustment rather than just guess at what might solve a problem.[13]

That idea that a manager/supervisor should "be among the team" is sometimes called "management by walking around"—MBWA for short. *The India Times* defined it beautifully:

MBWA basically refers to managers spending some part of their time listening to problems and ideas of their staff, while wandering around an office or plant.

Management by Walking Around is a term coined by management guru Tom Peters … [who] noticed that good managers tend to communicate a lot better with their team. And they do that in informal ways, like just hanging around in the office and chatting with them, rather than having formal interaction sessions in their cabins or boardrooms. …

The idea of this practice is to listen. You must

---

[13] Kimberlee Leonard, Houston, "What Is Performance Feedback?," *Chron.com*. Houston, TX: Houston Chronicle, Inc., 2018, https://smallbusiness.chron.com/performance-feedback-1882.html, accessed 5 July 2022.

also respond to ideas or problems voiced and take effective action about them.[14]

The Vice President at Hyatt Hotels, who gave me the great advice on handling the troublesome boss, used to say he practiced the butterfly version of management and leadership, checking in with his people and listening to them. The Managing Director of SRI and SRI Executive, Seamus McGardle, does the same. He is a remarkable leader, and friend, for countless reasons, but perhaps the most important is that he listens.

EXERCISE

So, now, at a little past half-way through our discussion, it's time to take a reading break to perform a test run. Feedback is a cornerstone principle of all success. "Performance measured is performance improved" has become a popular business maxim, for an obvious reason. Who can argue against it? As part of an organization, we have an obligation to that organization. That body has a right to hold us accountable for our performance. Is it not even more crucial that we hold ourselves accountable to ourselves for what we do? So, let's try it out.

Reread the "More of/Less of" section above and do that with yourself. (This doesn't have to be a comprehensive, full-body, self-examination. Pick just

---

[14] "What is 'Management By Walking Around'," *EconomicTimes. IndiaTimes.com, The Economic Times*. New Delhi, India: Times Internet Ltd., undated. https://economictimes.indiatimes.com/ definition/management-by-walking-around, accessed 5 July 2022.

one or two aspects of your life and ask yourself some serious questions then listen—really listen—to the answers.)

- What could I do more of to be a better workmate, partner, listener?
- And what might I do less of?
- If I was a co-worker evaluating me, what qualities would make me really appreciate associating with me?
- What do I need to feel content?

Now, sit down with a workmate, partner, close friend or relative—someone with whom you have a long history and high level of trust. Have them review the "More of/Less of" section, or even better, this whole chapter. You pick an aspect or two of your life for him or her to examine and have that person pick an aspect or two of his or her life for you to examine.

Like any skill, soliciting and obtaining quality feedback takes time to really develop and requires practice to maintain proficiency.

3. Plan Multiple Paths to Success

This feedback exercise is an example of a crucial conversation, and such dialogues require planning. My beloved, departed mother, Jo, would always say, "Imagine the worst that can happen. Plan for it, then everything else that can happen is better. After you do that plan, put it away and make a plan for a better-than-bad outcome. Then plan for the very best outcome you could have."

THINK THROUGH HOW TO HANDLE A CRUCIAL CONVERSATION

First, they're not chit-chat about the weather. Coined by a group of researchers at the turn of the century, "crucial conversations" refers to interactions of "high stakes, differing views, and strong emotions."[15] These terms are relative. A high-stakes subject to one person might be chit-chat to another. In fact, to a farmer, the weather—such as how to deal with a drought—is a very high stakes conversation. Likewise, some people are raised to never show emotion in public. To them, any display of anger or embarrassment or other feelings would be considered strong emotions.

Second, they're so rarely conducted successfully via text, email, or chat apps, that such a plan isn't worth considering. Crucial conversations need the human connection so that the participants can see, hear, and judge voice tone and inflexion; body language, like eye contact and posture; and everything else. Information is generally transmitted by the words we use, but the interpretation of data is very much affected by body language. Researchers have estimated that anywhere from 55 to 90 percent of communication is nonverbal. They add that, if there's an inconsistency between the attitudes conveyed by word and those conveyed by posture, posture will be, in almost every situation, the more convincing.

---

[15] Kerry Patterson, Joseph Grenny, Ron McMillan & Al Switzler, *Crucial Conversations: Tools for Talking When Stakes are High*. New York: McGraw-Hill Education, 2002

Finally, as the stakes rise higher, the views differ more widely, and emotions run stronger, consideration of the other person's feelings become more vital. For example, when bad news must be discussed, such as a project failure or a reduction in workforce, the recipients of that news deserve a face-to-face meeting, whether live or via satellite, not by email or text. It is simply a show of respect and professional courtesy. You don't want to burn bridges, make enemies, force someone to lose *face*, be humiliated, or suffer unnecessarily.

EVERYBODY'S GOT A PLAN A

Very few people actually see Plan A come to fruition. Good leaders always create a Plan B, a Plan C, and maybe several more if they think things could really go sideways. Look as objectively as you can at an upcoming crucial conversation and plan various scenarios in advance of those conversations to form a path to success.

Consider the following:

- What is your goal for the conversation? What goals might the other participants have?
- What is the relationship among the participants?
- What individual strengths, weaknesses, or other factors could affect the conversation?
- What outside influences may affect the conversation?
- What do you know about the situation? What do you think you know? What are you sure you don't know?

- Who is affected by the conversation's outcome? Positively or negatively?

Final Thought

Like so many other topics we've reviewed here, each individual person and individual situation will require a different level of crucial conversation planning. Practice will give you the tools to judge the level of "crucial" in any potential conversation.

4. Get in the Game

Many people have an unconscious, destructive habit. Either they ignore important issues or they minimise or devalue things that are important to other people and, essentially, dismiss those things. Both are tactics used by people who fear contention and do their utmost to avoid it. This is another habit you should be looking for in yourself and proactively working to eliminate. Contention happens and pretending it doesn't or avoiding it only makes it worse. As you get to know your teammates, it becomes easier to see their perspective and what you can do to accommodate their views without conflict. Sometimes, however, their priorities, which drive their perspective, are not so obvious.

As children, our needs are simple, and our attention span usually very short. Children need food, warmth, and security, and tend to focus on whatever catches their attention in a given moment.

As we grow, most people become increasingly (and surprisingly) complex. We don't always display our priorities in public. We develop deeply held beliefs that we cannot be moved from, such as religious or political views, which are, generally, not appropriate for workplace discussion. Sometimes, adults want what we want with childish passion.

In your scenario planning and in those crucial conversations, your head and your heart need to be focused on that conversation, its origins, processes, and ramifications. A crucial conversation requires commitment in preparation and execution.

Show Up

Zig Ziglar, the American author and motivational speaker, famously said, "If you're in something, get in it; if not, get out of it."[16] When you meet someone for a crucial conversation, that person and that subject become your top priority for those moments. Showing up is more than just walking into the room and shutting the door. It's leaving your phone at your desk or turning it off. It's telling your teammates that you are not to be disturbed unless the building catches fire. Focus your mind and attention on the business of the meeting. Develop the habit of recognizing and rejecting distractions like:

- Fleeting thoughts, such as "I need to pay the utility bills when I get home tonight" or "What should I do for lunch?" or "Did my friend text me back yet?" while looking at your phone.

---

[16] An often-repeated phrase in his public speeches.

- Topics you could discuss with the other partici-pants—called "chit-chat," "fluff," or "squirrels," among other things—that might be amusing, entertaining, or interesting, but distract from the goals of the meeting.
- Rehashing parts of the conversation that have already been decided.

"Showing up" is discipline and respect.

Slow Down

One of humanity's worst bad habits is our "need" to eliminate dead space. The awkward silences that arise every few minutes in normal discussions are disconcerting, but that's casual conversation—no harm, no problem if nothing life-changing gets said or not. A few seconds of thoughtful silence that arise between a comment and a response can be vital to the success of a crucial conversation because, by their nature, a crucial conversation—such as my interview with the hiring authority at DFID—can be truly life-changing.

- First, that moment of silence has other participants thinking, "You didn't spend the time I was speaking thinking about your response, you spent it really listening." That gains *face* and builds trust.
- Second, it gives you time to formulate a **proactive** response instead of offering a **reactive**, knee-jerk response.
- Finally, everybody's heard the phrase "rush to judgment." That's the fastest way to end

a crucial conversation without solving the problem. If you've set enough time to have and conclude a crucial conversation, then take that time. If not, then end when you must end and schedule more time to revisit the issues when you both can again devote your full attention to the subject.

We're all busy; we all have many roles to play and responsibilities to fulfill. Success comes more often to those who can place each role or responsibility in a box, take it out in its turn, and leave it alone when it is not.

TUNE IN

By showing up and slowing down, you show the other person that you're paying attention. You don't have to agree with everything others say, but you have to give them voice. As you do, you will, hopefully, come to a meeting of the minds—an understanding that this solution will meet the needs of all concerned and you all can proceed toward that solution with a clear conscience.

You can do more. As noted, I'm somewhere between an agnostic and an atheist, I don't know how the universe works and don't worry about it. But I recognize that any of us (maybe all of us) can be smarter and more aware than we are. We don't always have to be satisfied with a solution that meet the needs of all concerned. Sometimes, we can make a miracle. We can be brilliant, see what has never been seen before and make it happen. We can truly innovate, by working together.

For centuries it's been known that horses, though highly intelligent, really don't understand arithmetic. A single Belgian draft horse, for example, can pull a wagon and load totaling about 8,000 pounds. Simple math says that two Belgians should be able to pull twice that amount, a load of 16,000 pounds. Curiously, no one has ever been able to convince the horses of this elementary mathematical truth. Two Belgian drafts can, in fact, pull a load totaling 24,000 pounds. What does that say about working together?

Synergy, meaning "the whole is greater than the sum of the parts," is an undisputed fact. Somehow, a team, working together, can do more, accomplish more, be more than any individual or random group of individuals. It isn't automatic. It takes work. It requires us to build a team of the right people with the right skill sets and attitudes. My team at SRI, for example, doesn't need an architect. We learn, usually by trial and error, who is right to make the most perfect-as-possible blend of personalities and talents to accomplish great things.

5. SEE THE DIFFERENCES IN WHAT MOTIVATES TEAM MEMBERS

We hear this term a lot, but what, precisely, is "motivation"? Among its synonyms are catalyst, desire, drive, hunger, inducement, persuasion, spur, wish.[17] Hyrum Smith, Stephen Covey's co-founder at Franklin-Covey, called it the "fire in the belly" and often told his people that, as long as you have that fire, you keep

---

[17] "Motivation," *Thesaurus.com*, accessed 5 July 2022.

going. It's the internal feeling that pushes us to achieve whatever it is that we're after. Those achievements naturally make us feel more competent (and, therefore, less prone to imposter syndrome), less prone to stress in general, and they reduce our hesitation to take on future projects. On the other side, failures reduce our self-confidence, make us feel less competent (and more prone to imposter syndrome), contribute to increased stress, and may reduce our willingness to complete (or even to compete for) future projects.

So, how does one get motivated to accomplish a long list of tasks or a single large project? In coaching, I talk with people about this all the time. I hear things like, "I want to do A, B, and C. So, I'm going to jump on that, but I've got to do D, E, and F as well, and I don't really want to jump anywhere near them."

My responses are along these lines: "What can we do with that to get you motivated? Can we break it up, divide those projects into smaller pieces and share them with others?" "Can we find a part of it that you would enjoy? Would that encourage you enough to take it on with some measure of enthusiasm?"

Some people say, "I can get into this part of it, which I like. That'll get me on the road to do the rest." It's inertia. Once we get moving, it's easier to continue moving. Dividing a project into manageable portions also contributes. Saying, for example, "I'll do 100 sit ups every day," is a real challenge, especially when starting out. If you begin each morning by doing 10 before breakfast them commit to do another 10 by lunch then commit to doing another ten before midafternoon, etc., you'll eventually find yourself doing 100 daily with ease. You'll certainly be more likely than if you wake up every day and demand that you do 100 sit ups before breakfast!

Others like to tackle the hardest part first. Some people get motivated by doing the "heavy lifting" because, after that, the rest feels more like a long, easy slide to the finish line. This is something I was brought up to do by my father: attack the toughest part of the job first. If I was moving into a new apartment, what's the biggest, most difficult piece? It's the sofa or the double bed or something of equal size. Do that first and the rest feels easy by comparison.

Still others go the opposite direction, tackling the simplest aspects of the job first, getting a little success in hand so that, when tough times come, they can say, "I've come this far, I'm not going to see that effort wasted."

6. Assume the Right to Mirror Confidence

Assume means both "to take for granted or without proof" and "to take upon oneself."[18] Assuming the right to mirror confidence does both.

Almost a century ago, "Mahatma" Gandhi elaborated:

> Nor do I believe in inequalities between human beings. We are all absolutely equal. But equality is of the souls and not the bodies. Hence, it is a mental state. We need to think of, and to assert, equality because we see great inequality in the

---

[18] "Assume," *Dictionary.com*, accessed 5 July 2022.

physical world. We have to realize equality in the midst of this apparent external inequality. Assumption of superiority by any person over any other is a sin against God and man.[19]

Gandhi knew his words didn't reflect the reality of his times. Racial, ethnic, gender, and other prejudices existed then and continue to exist worldwide in some minds today.

The wiser among us take this as a challenge to overcome them. Despite all the advances women have made in their societies, more needs to be done. Gandhi wasn't lying in his statement, he was dreaming of a world where it would be true. The dream is the beginning of the reality.

Assuming the right to mirror confidence and, ultimately, to be confident, is the path to success. It is, in a real sense, the victory. If you, as an individual woman:

- Think about how your role models confidence and ask yourself, "How would s/he handle this situation?"
- Mirror the actions that follow from that attitude.
- Respond to others as if you already have the confidence you seek.
- Repeat this cycle until the act becomes a habit, second nature, an automatic response to any situation.

---

[19] Mohandas Karamchad "Mahatma" Gandhi, *Young India*. New York: B.W. Huebsch, Inc., 1923.

You become the confident woman you should be—the act becomes the persona. You win.

7. BE A ROLE MODEL FOR OTHER WOMEN

This is probably something you may be before you know you are. It may be that it happens naturally, organically, spontaneously by practicing these habits. That is, other women will see you as you've seen your role models and they will mirror you as you mirrored those who went before.

In many cases, it will be something you *do*:

- Look around you, see who needs coaching or mentoring or just a little encouragement.
- Adopt some obvious up-and-comers and some obvious strugglers as protégés.
- Coach and mentor them, by example and by educating them in how the system works.
- Encourage them to pay-it-forward by assisting those who follow them.

It's not likely that the Bible's Garden of Eden or Panem from Suzanne Collins' *The Hunger Games*—or any other literary utopias ever conceived—will actually happen. But we don't need to change the whole world, we just need to make the best of our little part of that world—and that is, definitely, something you can do.

CHAPTER 8

PIVOTAL PEOPLE, PIVOTAL MOMENTS

I never LOSE, I either WIN or LEARN.

—Nelson Mandela

INTRODUCTION — LOOKING FOR AN ISLAND

We left Kathmandu, Nepal, and spent the night in the town of Pokhara among the Himalayan foothills. Early the next morning, our rickety little aircraft took off and wove through the mountains to Jomsom, which lies north of Pokhara in the Mustang district and is the main gateway to Upper Mustang in Nepal, on the border with Tibet. Mount Everest is in the distance, snow covered, hiding its fury in the peaceful stillness from afar, breathtakingly beautiful. Jomsum sits south of the village of Kagbeni, a Tibetan-influenced village filled with prayer wheels, chortens, traditional Buddhist monuments, and a Buddhist monastery.

After we settled in at the sparse guesthouse, we walked through breathtaking mountain paths each morning, returning to the guesthouse by mid-day, to play cards and wait. The trail passing through Jomsom follows the Kali Gandaki River which forms the deepest ravine on the planet with the Annapurna Mountain range on one side. The Kali Gendaki freezes during winter and flows with rainwater and melting snow in summer.

With its diverse landscape, the area around Jomsom has remarkable scenery—the rocky cliffs and high peaks of the Himalayas, but without much greenery in this season. We heard that each spring brings fields of bright rhododendrons, but it was somewhat bleak that late in Autumn and getting colder by the day, with winter settling in soon.

The culture in Jomsom was a rich combination of Hinduism and Tibetan Buddhism and we heard the soft sounds of drums and chanting around each mountain trail during our morning walks. Each morning, we passed trekkers with huge packs on their backs, who spent their nights on the mountain to achieve their life's dream—reaching the summit of the world's highest peak—but we were not there for that. We were waiting for a child. My sister had come to adopt a Nepali baby.

It was late October and, if we didn't achieve success soon and get back down the mountain to Kathmandu, the snows would lock us in until April. The tiny planes weren't be able to manoeuvre through the air pockets, winds, and myriad dangers of the Himalayan winter. Soon, the little prop jobs that transported trekkers in and out of the nearby base camp wouldn't be able navigate the treacherous mountains they must glide through to get us back to Kathmandu then to the outside world. After a few more days, they wouldn't be able to take off in the increasing winds. We'd have been snowed in—frozen here in the huts, like Jomsom's natives are for six months every year.

We'd learned from the trekkers that some of them never resume their climb past Jomson because the altitude can stop you dead in your tracks before the mountain does. We believed them and we awoke early each day while we waited to complete our walk because, by noon, the storms and winds were coming in so powerfully they could literally blow you off your feet.

Our refuge was this small guesthouse room with three cots—one for my sister, Becky, who'd been unable to have her own child and was desperate to be a mother; one for my brother, a doctor; and one for me. It had one toilet that regularly gets so clogged we had to manually unclog it.

When Becky got a call, about a month before, that there was a baby available for adoption in the mountains of the Himalayas, she didn't hesitate. She pleaded with me to come from London to meet her in Kathmandu and make the rest of the journey with her to find this child. She thought I'd know something about babies because I was then a young mother of two. She asked Dan to come from El Salvador where he was practicing medicine at the time. She was wise to think a doctor might be handy on this trip. Even though we weren't trekking, this was a dangerous trip for us and for the child, if we found her, and dangerous to get a poor, malnourished child legally out of these treacherous mountain passes, back to Kathmandu, out of Nepal, and into the to the USA where Becky lived. So, we waited.

Our adoption agency contact was Laksman, the English nickname for the Nepali man who was the liaison for the adoption. He floated in and out of the villages in these mountains seeking babies for adoption. It had been almost three weeks since Laksman told us that a very poor Nepali woman would come down through the mountain pass, so we watched every day. He said she'd bring the baby my sister might be able to adopt. The fear and sadness in my sister's eyes grew more apparent every hour as the snowline daily descended, coming closer to shutting us in. Our window of opportunity shrank, it seemed, by the hour and she was being crushed by the idea that she'd never be a mother. She'd been to Romania the year before and had, sadly, returned with no child, motherhood again out of her reach.

Each morning, the air had been crisp and still but, by noon, the wind and sand had whipped into a storm. Now, sand was being replaced by snow. The storms fogged the skies and our minds, yet we peered through squinting eyes each morning at the mountain pass entrance, hoping for the child to magically appear. My own children, then aged 2 and 4, had been left behind in the UK for a month with their father. He cared for them while I accompanied my sister on this remote and rugged trek to find her a family, hoping it wouldn't be another heart-breaking wild goose chase. We prayed to Buddha that we wouldn't leave empty handed. On the last morning, deflated of all hope, we wordlessly started packing our meagre gear.

But that last morning, as we squinted toward the path's entrance through the daily storm, the miracle happened. In the middle of that meteorological mess, we saw a tiny woman lead a donkey along the snowy mountain pass. Her shoes were tied round the tops of her feet but had no soles, she was effectively barefoot. There was a baby strapped across the back of the donkey. Laksman, who was there to say a sad goodbye, suddenly cried out and pointed to her. Through the flurries, he ran out to greet her in Nepalese, and helped her untie the child from the donkey, bringing them both inside the guesthouse, to the warmth near the fire.

We offered this diminutive but weathered mother hard-boiled eggs and tea, which she almost inhaled, eating ravenously because she was, literally, starving.

Our interpreter asked her if we could hold the tiny child. As Becky took the baby, my heart nearly broke in relief for them both. We were told the baby was 18 months old, but she couldn't walk because, each day, her mother had to work the fields for 12 hours. Every morning at dawn, the baby, called Karsang, had been tied into a wrap on her mother's back to be carried to a huge flat rock next to the field. Karsang spent her days sleeping on the rock or tied to her mother's back while she worked, bent in the fields. Karsang had never used her legs. The baby was fragile but beautiful and I could see the relief and joy in my sister's face as she finally saw her yearned-for future unfold before her. Now, she could be what she wanted to be for 40 years—a mother. Karsang's mother bravely told Laksman that she was too poor to care for her child and she wanted her baby to have a better life. Becky knew that growing up in Denver, Colorado, with her adoptive mother wouldn't be easy with a name like

Karsang, so, this baby, my new niece, was reborn that day as Kara.

Kara's clothes were sewn on around her, with a slit in the back of the pants. Changing clothes was, in this culture, for rich people. The poorest of the poor couldn't afford the luxury of several sets of clothing, so the scraps were simply sewn on until a child grew so much that she burst out of them—by which time, hopefully, her mother would've saved another scrap to be stitched on to expand the rags that were all the wardrobe this child had ever had.

Becky and Dan sat with Laksman, Kara's birth mother (who made her mark, an X) and a local official who also had to sign the agreement so Kara could be taken. I was tasked with gently cutting the sewn-on clothes off the crying baby, then trying to bathe her and wash her matted hair. While I did so, I saw my own tears gently dripping into the tub of water. Kara cried because of the shock of warm water and strange hands, but I cried for sheer happiness for my new niece and her new mother. And, admittedly, some sadness for Kara's birth mother to watch her child go forever.

I realised much later that, during this month of my life, I saw extraordinary strength—pivotal people and pivotal moments. Kara's birth mother was a pivotal person in my life. To know the deep, heart-wrenching love for your child as I do, then see a mother who trekked across a mountain range in sole-less shoes and freezing storms to give her child a better life was an enormous act of love. My sister took another huge risk of heartbreak to go halfway around the planet in the hope she'd find Kara and bring her home. Dan and I were only background players in this drama, but we learned so much from them both in taking chances, facing potential heartbreak, and finally reaping the benefits of those risks. I learned then, that the island might not always be in sight, but sometimes, you just have to jump into the water and start swimming because you have faith that the island will appear.

THE PANDEMIC, THE GREAT RESIGNATION AND THE GREAT RE-EVALUATION

Over the last year, 2021 through mid-2022, there's been a lot of public discussion about "the Great Resignation." The media got wind of that term and adopted it, giving it such wide publicity that it's become part of the common jargon. But the term isn't entirely accurate. It suggests that everyone's just quitting their jobs, going off-grid and living in the fields eating beansprouts. That is far from the truth. People aren't joining the unemployment rolls by the millions, many are changing jobs, even industries. The pandemic and our lockdowns gave space to people around the world to reevaluate how they want to live their time on Earth. Faced with real threats of illness or death tends to focus the mind.

Since March 2020, people have been increasingly thinking about their mortality. Yes, there is a correlation between age and mortality. In any generation, as people get older, their health breaks down in new and unpleasant ways, they tend to get sick and, eventually, leave the Earth. Death is obviously closer with each passing decade. However, with constant news coverage hammering us with talk of a global pandemic, war, economic threats, and with death via new viral mutations reaching out to many young, otherwise healthy people, the younger generations, too, have had moments where their mortality stared them in the face.

During 2020 and 2021, millions of people asked, for the first time, one of the ultimate questions of life: "I have a finite time here, there's a virus that might just end me. How am I going to spend what time remains?" As 2021 became 2022, the survivors started asking new questions, "Is this job really what I want to be doing? Is this thing that I'm doing with these people in this organization what I want to do for the next 20 or 30 years? Do I feel good about it? Am I making a difference?"

COVID-related job dissatisfaction is one of the direct causes of the Great Resignation. During the lockdown, people had fewer activities, so more time to think about serious issues. With little kids at home, many probably had less personal time, but time with children probably led many to be introspective. With fewer distractions, many seem to have taken time to reorganize their lives a bit and consider how they want their lives to be spent when the world opened up again.

All that, I believe, made people more self-aware and more interested in taking the long view of their lives. Self-help books have enjoyed a robust growth over the past decade, up 11 percent per year from 2013 to 2019, but sales jumped 25 percent in 2021 alone.[20, 21] More people started asking, "How should I spend my time? Who am I as a person? How can I be better as a person? How can I go from the past into the direction that I want?"

The Great Resignation wasn't a resignation, it was a **Great Re-Evaluation**. We saw record numbers of people changing jobs. Some said, "I'm quitting. I'm taking a hiatus to think about what I want out of life." Many others said, "I don't have to simply keep going through the routine that I've been going through. It isn't fulfilling me, so, I'm going to do something different, something that excites my soul, instead of just making my banker happy."

In the long run, I think this will be good for those individuals and for the human race as a whole.

EI/EQ Revisited

Recently, the Secretary General of a major UN organization and I discussed future hires. His was a scientific agency, so most of his employees were scientists, but

---

[20] Dennis Pierce, "Self-Help Books Fill a Burgeoning Need," *LibraryJournal.com*. New York City: Library Journal, Inc., 9 March 2021. https://www.libraryjournal.com/story/self-help-books-fill-a-burgeoning-need#:~:text=The%20self%2Dhelp%20industry%20has,period%2C%20from%2030%2C897%20to%2085,253, accessed 29 June 2022).

[21] Jim Milliot, "Self-Improvement Boom Sets Book Sales Off on Fast Start in 2021," *PublishersWeekly.com*. New York City: PWxyz, LLC, 14 January 2021. https://www.publishersweekly.com/pw/by-topic/industry-news/bookselling/article/85316-book-sales-get-off-to-fast-start.html, (accessed 29 June 2022).

professional competence wasn't his only criteria. He said, specifically, "I can find all the great scientists in the world." He was hiring 20 new scientists at that time, all of them top-level experts in their disciplines. The SG told me, "I can find lots of great scientists, but if they can't deal with other people, aren't aware of what's going on, and don't have a high level of emotional intelligence or EQ, and therefore aren't good leadership potential, I don't want them." I really admire this SG for his stance on the value of EQ.

Although that agency, like many public sector entities, had its communications and media people and that whole science machine was humming, the switched-on Secretary General recognized that people skills are as important as technical skills.

I was extremely pleased to hear this, because I believe in it so much. I have huge respect for scientists, both my father and brother work in medicine, and I'm a behavioral scientist. But typically, scientific training doesn't include emotional intelligence/emotional quotient (EI/EQ) skills. Unfortunately, too often, scientists are selected for jobs, leadership posts, speaking engagements, and everything else, based solely on technical credentials—the degrees behind their name, the papers they've published, the interviews they've already given. Despite a decade or more of university, plus ongoing training, they never get taught the necessity of developing their EI/EQ. So, I was really happy to hear that this influential executive understood their value.

The SG's attitude becomes less unique day by day. Many business and government leaders are getting the message and adopting job requirements which include high emotional intelligence as vital for the role. As more workers continue to abandon the "great career" of huge salaries and bonuses, extensive perks, and pure-profit motives, and continue seeking employment that matches their ideals, they need to be prepared with EI/EQ and other skills in addition to their technical skills.

"But I've never heard of or been trained in EI/EQ!" may become a common fear in the job-hunting community. Guess what—you can learn it.

TALENTS OR SKILLS?

There are those among us who seem to be "born to lead," like a piano or math prodigy. They seem to naturally understand EI/EQ and practice the skills of good leadership. This has caused some to assume that leadership is a talent with which we're born, or not, and that's the end of the story.

In fact, most leadership studies have concluded you don't have to be "born to lead." I'm certain that the same applies equally to, if not more so with, EI/EQ. We've all heard someone ask, "Can you sing?" or something similar. The answer is (or should be), "Yes." Everybody can sing. Few of us do it well enough to get paid for it, most of us wouldn't even qualify for the church or community choir, but all of us can do it and all of us can be taught to do it better.

In this respect, there's no difference between leadership and singing, writing, dancing, any other art or any technical skill. We can all do it and we can all learn to do it better. If you can learn, you can lead.

Likewise, all of us have what's called a "gut instinct" and a conscience. Most of us instinctively know right from wrong. All of us know how we want to be treated. You're a good leader if you:

- Realize that you are a leader—of your own life if nothing else.
- Follow your gut instinct. Trust yourself.
- Treat others as well as you feel you should be treated.

That's all the leadership and EI/EQ you need to start. From there, as you gain more experience, as you seek out and take advantage of the many books, seminars, college/university classes, and professional coaching/mentoring opportunities, your inborn talents can be honed onto fine skills, but you must use your head, heart and hands. In emotional intelligence assessment, we call this reality testing—do you use everything that is available to you, from data, instinct, team power, or advice? When you realize the power of the team, you are practicing generative leadership.

In a 2022 publication, Boston Consulting Group summarizes *The Power of the Head, Heart, and Hands*:

Leading with the head involves not only reimagining your company's products and services but also leading the way across organizations to reinvent industries. Generative leaders cultivate and reward creative thinking in their teams. And they pursue new technologies and ideas that once seemed impossible.

Leading with the heart means seeking to inspire and enrich the human experience by building great cultures and workplaces where people can do their best work. Generative leaders invest deeply in relationships, especially during difficult times. They prioritize coaching and development to help people realize their full potential, and they celebrate success, learning, and progress.

Leading with the hands includes creating high-functioning, empowered, and cross-functional supercharged teams that execute and innovate with agility. These teams can move quickly and in unison, anticipating where the ball will land rather than focusing on where it is in the moment. They adapt to changing conditions. Generative leaders build resilience in their teams by ensuring a balance between sprints and recovery.

Putting Generative Leadership into Practice

Francesco Starace, CEO of Italian utility Enel, is a great example of a generative leader. In order to move the company into renewable energy, he made a number of remarkably bold moves. He encouraged team members to spend 20% of their time on innovative projects, introduced a "my best failure" initiative to promote creativity and encourage risk taking, and launched a crowdsourcing platform that allows outsiders to propose solutions to different innovation challenges.

This kind of generative approach advocates and celebrates team leadership, not heroic individual leaders. Six years after launching this program of reinvention, Enel became the world's largest supplier of renewable energy—and increased its market value by 2.6 times.

All good leaders develop an instinct that identifies values in people, recognizes innovation, and ideas that might have merit—minor players who can grow into major contributors and projects that can best forward the group's goals.

The culture in which you spend 30 years with the same company then retire with a dinner and a gold watch is gone. A recent article from IT recruiter Apollo Technical states[22]:

You often hear about people changing careers an average of seven times during their lifetime. The problem is there is no actual data to back it up. [However] ... It is estimated that most

---

[22] Jean-Michel Caye, Jim Hemerling, Deborah Lovich, Marie Humblot-Ferrero, Fanny Potier, and Robert Werner, "Why the World Needs Generative Leaders," *BCG.com*. Boston: Boston Consulting Group, March 17, 2022. https://www.bcg.com/publications/2022/all-about-generative-leadership-and-its-benefits, accessed 30 June 2022.

people will have 12 jobs during their lives. In the last year, 32% of those 25 to 44 have considered a career change. Since starting their first job after college, 29% of people have completely changed fields.[23]

The rate of job change among the Millennial and Gen-Z generations is much higher than Baby Boomers and Gen-Xers.[24] Fifty-three percent of the younger generation compared to only 35 percent of the older gens are considering changing jobs this year, according to the *Microsoft 2022 Work Trend Index*.[25] Studies also indicate increasing numbers of Gen-Zers opting into the gig economy, working one gig at a time. Perhaps each gig is a pivotal moment for that person.

So, why do people change careers?

- Increased salary, responsibility, rank, or opportunity

[23] "17 Remarkable Career Change Statistics To Know," *ApolloTechnical.com*, Smyrna GA: Apollo Technical, 19 March 2022. https://www.apollotechnical.com/career-change-statistics/, accessed 30 June 2022.

[24] "Baby Boomers" is an official designation by the United States Census Bureau, referring to the notable surge in births following World War II from 1946 thru 1964. Unofficially, later generations received nicknames for convenience in comparison: Gen-X (1965-1980), Millennials (1981-1996) and Gen-Z or "Zoomers" (1997-2012). Among demographic researchers, there are some variations in these designations and timetables.

[25] Yaël Bizouati-Kennedy, "52% of Gen Z and Millennial Employees Willing to Change Jobs This Year," *GoBankingRates.com*. El Segundo, CA: ConsumerTrack, Inc., (undated). https://www.gobankingrates.com/money/jobs/gen-z-millennial-employees-willing-to-change-jobs-this-year/, accessed 7 July 2022.

- Changing philosophy and goals (of the worker or the company)
- Dissatisfaction with leadership at the current company
- Desire to have greater flexibility in work
- Unsatisfied with one's current career
- Curious about the world
- Motivated by change and new challenges
- Prefer the non-traditional work-from-home options heavily promoted during the pandemic

Among countless other reasons.

Conclusion

I sit here thinking, sinking
Into a puddle
The rain is falling, then you give me your hand.
The rain goes away
The pain goes away.
Don't let me go.

— J. Simmons

The Precipice

My son's eyes are rolling back in his head. He's barely conscious and his emaciated 6-foot frame is dangling off the edge of the scrappy hospital bed in a back street clinic with dirt floors on the periphery of Ouagadougou. Have you ever heard of that place? I hadn't either, until we were transferred there, the capital city of Burkina Faso, the poorest country in Africa. We live in a decent house, behind tall metal gates. All ex-patriate white people do because we are funded by rich Aid agencies. The gates to the world outside open to dirt streets, flowing sewers and swarms of starving children while we are inside the compound with a cook, a driver, a pool cleaner, and a man who irons all day, including my underwear. (This makes me very uncomfortable.) We employ as many as we can so they can feed their families. When they go home, they go to mud huts that wash away every year in the monsoons.

Harrison has typhoid and malaria simultaneously—again. When we arrived in Ouagadougou a few months ago, Harrison carried 90 kilos on his 6-foot 3-inch frame. But, now, he's lost 20 kilos and his blonde, floppy hair sticks to the damp sweat of his 16-year-old forehead.

He needs fluids urgently, dehydrated from all the vomiting and diarrhea, and I've rushed him here to the ramshackle clinic. There's nowhere else to rush him because, I know from working in health settings in developing countries for years, that more people die of dehydration than anything else. Maybe the next one could be my son. This morning Harrison worsened, I panicked, then called the Belgian Missionary doctor again. He finally arrived through the gates to see Harrison on our screened porch, the Doctor was sweating profusely at 9.00 AM from the heat, already 45-degrees Celsius, and asked for something to drink. I offered water but he insisted on beer and shot it back in seconds before feeling Harrison's sopping brow again. He looked from his own glassy eyes into Harrison's sunken ones. He proclaimed, "Harrison's situation needs urgent medical attention and I need another beer."

THE COLOR OF HELP

Now, at the clinic, I am terrified my son will die. He will not respond to the medicines given orally, we cannot stop the weight loss, whatever antibodies Burkina Faso has to offer, they are finding unwelcome hosts in my son's body. It is my moment of truth to figure out how to save him, but I am lost. I am also flooded with everything else my life is handing me. My business idea cannot be realized here, and my daughter has a chronic illness but is alone in the USA. She can't visit here because her disease won't allow her to have the live vaccines for yellow fever which are mandatory to enter Burkina Faso. My husband is doing everything to be a good development professional, a good husband, a good stepfather, but he must make the hour-long trek though these filthy streets twice a day to work for the Dutch Development Agency on the other side of Ouagadougou. Everything is failing. I need to find a lifeline. I didn't know the lifeline was inside me all the time.

WHY GUT MATTERS

At the remote clinic, if they don't get intravenous fluids into Harrison very soon, he will lose consciousness. Everyone speaks French here, no English is spoken, yet I had agreed to bring my son here without being able to utter a word, even to the workers in the house. Why did I do that?

The clinic has enlisted a young white female Aid worker to try to put a needle intravenously into Harrison's long, floppy arm. Her ungloved hands are shaking as the clinic staff surround her and shout to get his vein. The shouting is all in Burkinabe French, which I don't speak or understand. I forget in my panicked state, that the girl is Scandinavian, so she probably speaks some English.

The terrified trainee repeatedly jabs a needle into Harrison's arm, missing, and they are both violently shaking as his blood drips onto the dirt floor. I am not calm, but pleading in English, "We need a **doctor** not an inexperienced volunteer!" while again trying to ring my French speaking husband, to come. He is in meetings across town, but it's a city of a million heaving poor people, all dirt roads, dust, horse carts, motos and chaos. I finally get his office on the phone. They will tell him to come. I am losing control, which is not usual for me. I finally get my wits in order and realize that I must get Harrison to the airport, onto a plane and if he lives, we will fly out of this purgatory forever.

I am pleading with the cowering medical staff, doing nothing but shouting at the white girl, who is as frightened as any one I have ever seen. I feel her trauma and want to help her, but I can't, nor can I understand why they can't get someone to insert the IV into my dying son's arm. There are very good Burkinabe nurses in this clinic. They have done the same for Harrison before—when he was less critical than today—and for me, when I had malaria. After each time Harrison has been sick, we stabilize him, send him to London to recover, he then returns, tries to stay here but is almost immediately ill again. Malaria and typhoid are the killers of West Africa that everyone knows so intimately.

Finally, my husband arrives, screaming up in the dusty wake made by our massive old clunker Aid-worker jeep. It is the only reliable car to have when you drive through floods, dirt tracks and cow dung every day. Tim comes in, takes complete control in perfect French, and immediately the terrified girl is asked to step away, as a young black Burkinabe male nurse who had been silent in the back of the pack comes forward. I recognize him as the man who had previously so adeptly inserted an IV in both Harrison and me in earlier days. I learn later that Tim has been told the young white girl is a new volunteer and was never trained to insert an IV. I am bewildered and furious.

Why are they just pulling the young male nurse into service now? But now is not the time to investigate, because the only thing that matters is getting the needle into my son so he can get the fluids that will keep him alive. The male nurse swiftly responds after the clinic manager shouts something shrill in French. He steps forward, takes the needle from the girl's shaking hands, reaffirms its connection to the drip, and tightens the tourniquet on Harrison's bicep, taps the vein and deftly inserts it. The needle is in the vein, the drip is turned full flow. Harrison becomes quiet and I hold his head in my lap. Harrison will live.

SHIFTING TOWARD BRAVERY

The drunken Belgian doctor is on his way, and only then, during the lull, does Tim tell me that the Scandinavian intern had no medical training ever. She was simply stabbing my son's arm with a needle because clinic staff told her to do it. She was the only white person in the clinic. The rest of the staff were too afraid to let the more skilled Burkinabe clinicians take the risk, until my husband came and insisted in French, and there was no way out for them. They could all see Harrison was very ill, near death, but a native black Burkinabe could never survive killing a rich, white boy. That would be their own death sentence. And a young woman, though white, because of her lack of and without confidence, could not exert her power and step away from a situation she had no business being in. I have instantly learned that there are forces beyond what I know and what I have seen and felt, and I must try to find them earlier so I can make better choices and be braver. I need to use my gut.

After Harrison is evacuated back to London, I feel there has been a mega-shift in me. I know I must be smarter and more courageous to seek and find alternative ways through life's challenges, whether they are personal or professional, but I somehow know that what I need is inside of me. How to find it and act on it? I need to find my true path.

I pondered this for most of a year, until we were transferred from the poorest country in the world, to one of the richest places on the planet, the South of France. My master's degree was done long ago, but I needed to learn more. Now, I needed to know how to harness the power inside me to speak out while still being my authentic self, how to give confidence to those to whom it did not naturally come, how to share knowledge with those without power to find their own power, their own success, their own true path.

My business idea, to help those from developing countries to realize their full potential, was forming in my mind. In France, it finally became a reality. I could use the developed world's advantages to empower women, both in developing and less-developed nations, and women everywhere who did not quite believe in their own abilities. I had a great education, but I realized that I had never had any formal training in the most essential aspects of life. The important things in life were not taught: how to be confident, how to survive heartbreak, how to really listen, how to call out wrong but stay kind, and most importantly, humility. I acknowledged my place in the world and the powerful advantages I had been given by being born white and well-off. I finally understood how to use these advantages to fully engage those born without them.

My long-term goal molded my short-term goal, and it happened in a day. Just before we left Ouagadougou, I was riding my bike on a dirt road, with the stench from open sewers lining the streets making me wretch while I rode. I was on my way to a French class in a mud hut. When I came home that day, Harrison said he had seen something disturbing. He showed a picture he had taken on his old Nokia phone—a rudimentary sign spray-painted on a shack near his school. It said, "Young Girls for Sale Here." Harrison was as repulsed as I was.

My business idea changed to a different plan: Talk to young women. Learn what they lived through. Find a way help them rise out of the condemned purgatory of being sold for sex or treated with subjugation. Change their beliefs about their own abilities.

There is a mantra in international development that is a universal truth. Education is the only way out of poverty and subjugation. I decided to learn, to teach, to listen more and to connect with role models who felt the same. As my goals shifted, my mind shifted, and my results started to become reality.

VivePoint is Born

In old English *vivepoint* means "continual change with perpetual improvement." With a remarkable friend, we started an organization to seek out, find, and coach women to find their own confidence and bravery. When women were able to take a professional step forward, we ran a mile in happiness.

There are still challenges and doubts, but there was a seminal moment for change as we built the idea of the business from our guts, and it felt like a calling. I became more brave, less fearful of failure and I learned that fear is motivating, stimulating, scary. In the moments I feel terrified, I try to remember I'm learning and to find what needs changing. We are still learning enormously, and we are teaching what we learn. We base every coaching and teaching session on seeking tough empathy. We coach them to identify their goals, targets, and dreams. Find them. Focus on them. Don't ever lose sight of them. Empathy means all those dreams involve other people. And always remember that every single person you see or pass on the street or speak to has a tragedy of their own, big or small. So, without empathy, we are nothing.

Now, VivePoint connects with women and men all over the world, coaching and mentoring toward confidence and using tough empathy as our gold standard. This is our mantra, our system of beliefs, that whatever we give will be given back to us in gratitude, in trust, in kindness and in human connection. More than I would have hoped, in this consulting work and through crucial conversations, we are told every day that we have changed someone's life, given them confidence, helped them find their true path. For this I will be forever grateful. This is my measurement of success. Money helps, but for me, it will never overcome the value of appreciation and being a catalyst for change.

I learned that, to be a leader did not only mean to have the big job, which I did, as a CEO of a leading healthcare organization working in 50 countries to address the problems of unsafe sex; as a sought-after executive search advisor, finding and hiring the heads of United Nations agencies; as a professional executive coach, advising world leaders to be even better leaders and better people. I've been fortunate to make the right connections at senior levels, which I continue to have and appreciate. However, most of all, I have the great joy of seeing the power in all people, whatever their place in the world.

Sometimes, I wonder if I should carry along the path I'm following or change, because ideas are always coming to me. I have monkey mind! But the gauge is my heart and my gut. I rely on gut and EI, not IQ. There are many people with a higher IQ than mine, I'm certain. But I'm proud to say that I always measure my success by those who say, "You changed my life because you believed in me and helped me find what I had inside." For every single person I coach and mentor, this is a primary tenant of success—improving your own emotional intelligence, your own heart, your own path.

In leading, caring makes you a leader who lasts. Not the Ph.D., not the reams of publications, not the bank account. It's the understanding of what tough empathy means: Drive toward your goals. Insist on results. See the potential in every person you meet.

When you do, your business will last and your heart will lead you. What more could you ask for?

POSTSCRIPT

Harrison recovered after three evacuations to the UK. Each time he bravely returned to Ouagadougou, but typhoid and malaria got him again and again. He went to Ouagadougou a privileged white, blond 15-year-old kid with too many clothes, gadgets, and advantages. He left there with one tee shirt, a ragged pair of shorts, flip flops, and his own mantra—to give, to love and to be a person who shares everything from shoes, clothes, and knowledge, to his heart. He will always be somewhere knocking mangoes off trees to feed poor kids who followed him home from school every day, just to germinate hope in them. And whatever grows in them, we will find it, and nurture it so they can grow strong and confident.

CHAPTER 9

PACKAGING YOURSELF FOR MAXIMUM IMPACT

It always seems impossible until it's done.

—Nelson Mandela

INTRODUCTION — REALITY CHECK

Every smart woman should have the Reality Check Buddy (RCB). This is the person to whom you can explain a circumstance or a problem or a situation in which you have a certain point of view but want to see what you may be missing. You may like or admire a lot of people, but the RCB is different. You must take time and think about who has the courage, confidence, and honesty to really tell you if they think you're missing something important, or they believe you are just wrong and should reconsider your position. Also, this is someone you must trust absolutely to keep everything in the strictest confidence. To give this kind of feedback requires a kind of unconditional respect for each other, so pick your RCB wisely and set out the terms of your reality check interactions.

I'm lucky. I've had an RCB, Pippa, for a very long time. I can ask her about a professional or personal situation or an event or dilemma and I know I'll get a straight answer from her on whether my view is sound and reasonable. Sometimes, she'll tell me I'm completely off-base and have missed something. She might explain a lateral perspective I didn't see or a spin-off problem I may not have considered. Sometimes, she'll say I've gotten it exactly right. Other times, it's a combination of both. I do the same for her, and we've never come away with hurt feelings if one says the other got it wrong or missed something, and we never feel that criticisms have been made. It helps that we're both trained coaches, but we weren't always. She's was a wonderful RCB when we went through our coaching certifications at different times. We share opinions, and we know it's just an opinion, though sometimes based on facts. Many times over many years this has helped us both enormously.

We also have an open policy, agreed between us when we started, that either of us can "use or lose" the information we share, without recrimination or regret. That means I can take her advice, keep and use what is authentically me, or ignore it, and she'll never take offense. It's very liberating to know you have an RCB and it's a great benefit to have such a person, one who's willing to be as honest as they must be to help you.

I have a difficult client, a senior member of an international development financial institution. He's not very high in EI/EQ, therefore, doesn't use much finesse when dealing with others. Remarkably, (and, frankly, irritatingly), he's in a talent management role in the bank, meaning he has the power to hire and fire for the bank, and contracts me (through the SRI agency) to lead senior headhunting searches for him. He's been quite curt and critical of me and my project staff several times, which I don't admire. I am happy to take feedback, but not groundless moaning. He is the client, but contrary to popular belief, I don't think the client is always right. I set boundaries—a line of behavioural acceptability that I adhere to because of my own self-respect and my insistence that others treat me and my team with respect.

After a few experiences with him being rude and punitive about small issues, I called my RCB and explained my situation to her. I didn't want to compromise the relationship with a client, but I was nearing my limit on his terse, rude verbal and written communication. I was fed up with him putting something or someone down unnecessarily. We talked about this behaviour being common with insecure individuals, a fact that didn't make it easier to bear. I was near to a point of writing him an email to say this behaviour and tone was unacceptable.

My RCB asked me some more particulars about him and the exchanges we previously had. She reminded me that writing is one-way communication and, in times of potential disagreement, texting or emailing is often the worst way to communicate. It can't be accompanied by tone of voice, as in phoning or body language, as in interviewing. Although words are important, many studies show we instinctively use tone and body language to communicate far more than words can ever convey alone. In fact, writing can be (and often is) easily misconstrued when stakes are high. My RCB asked me to define my desired end result.

Well, my first thought revolved around my banker client miraculously going **poof** and becoming a high-EQ, self-aware individual. That was not going to happen. So, my reality check became asking myself, "What might be possible to improve, if not completely fix, this uncomfortable situation?"

I told my RCB that I believed it might be possible to improve if I used my own EQ skills softly to see if we could improve our exchanges. She also suggested I wait until the next time it happened, so there was a clear pattern to refer to. We role-played this between us, but I did not have to wait long.

Just a few days after my discussion, it happened again and I decided to email him asking for a private chat when he had a minute. He agreed and I telephoned him, modulated my voice to be soft and explorational, telling him I felt our exchanges seemed strained to me and asked him if he thought we somehow had gotten off on the "wrong foot"?

Then I did what is so hard for so many: I waited, and kept my mouth shut.

He seemed confused, then said, "Well, no, I don't think so," which told me clearly, he was unaware of his own behaviour and demeanour. I asked him, "Is there anything about the way that I work with you that you would like to change?"

He said "No, I don't think so."

Then I offered, "Could we agree to be straightforward about needs, but not punitive in tone over email or calls?" I explained that I have a responsibility to my team, as I was sure he did to his, for them to maintain a high standard of respectful communications. To my surprise, he said "Well, yes, of course."

I thanked him for his time and we ended the call. He must've given the discussion some thought because, although he never turned into the politest of clients, he stopped the punitive words and surly tone he had been using. I was very grateful to my RCB, and to myself for listening to her.

Resumes or and Curricula Vitae (CVs)

There is a difference between a resume and a curriculum vitae, or "CV" for short.

A resume or CV, as we call it in Europe, is a summary of your work history, experiences, skills, and education. A resume that's too short, less than one page, might be ignored because the hiring authority will view the candidate as inexperienced. Unless it's an entry-level job, where a short resume is expected. Exceptionally long resumes may get rejected because the HR staff simply doesn't want to read them. It's their job to pick a half-dozen candidates (or fewer) to present to the hiring authority. If they get a dozen candidates, they have time to delve deeply into each one. A desirable job, however, might attract 200 resumes or more. In such cases, HR staff could refuse 195 of them and they may have the smallest excuse to refuse yours.

CVs need to do two things:

- Show all that you've accomplished, setting you apart from everyone else
- Demonstrate your assets, how you can meet the needs of the hiring organisation

THE PITCH AND THE INTERVIEW

A CV is a calling card. It's that first meeting with the prospective buyer and the product you're selling. That product is you.

You're not selling a mass-produced product to everybody whether they want it or not. You're not trying to discover or create some need in the buyer's mind that your product fills, then hand off the product, collect their money, and move on, never to meet again.

You're offering a unique item, yourself, and looking for a partnership situation between you and the company that satisfies your needs, and theirs. A CV, therefore, should be customized for each application, based on research into the company or organisation. You may think that's a lot of work and it is more work, but it's worthwhile. You've got to get in the organisation's mind:

- What are they looking for?
- What do they need?
- How do I fit into their plan and fill their needs?

- What's the culture? Will I blossom or wither in that garden?
- How can I help them solve their problems?

Fortunately, that's a lot easier these days, because you can find a wealth of information online. The organisation's annual reports and social media will often tell you everything you need to know about their history, strategy and results.

For example, among many of the organisations SRI Executive serves, you'd want to look at the 17 Sustainable Development Goals (SDGs) and the projects each organisation undertakes to reach those goals. In 2015, the UN General Assembly adopted these SDGs, emphasizing a holistic approach to sustainable development planetwide. Each UN agency and many of their international partners are focused on one or a few of these goals. Knowing exactly how this agency is oriented and where their resources will be expended makes it possible to tailor your CV to demonstrate how you can contribute to their vision and mission. The same is true of most large businesses.

When you get to the interview, you might then say, "I see you want to make progress in this particular area— women's empowerment in Southeast Asia. I have done some work in that area. Here's what I could do for you to help you reach your goals."

Or, perhaps, an industrial tractor manufacturer currently builds fossil-fueled vehicles, but they want to market a line of electric vehicles, eventually replacing the diesels completely. Alternative-fuel technology is not yet commercially viable in that arena. Assuming that the firm wants to hire long-term employees, they'll probably be looking for applicants who have fossil-fuel engineering skills and have or can acquire alternative-fuels skills. A prime candidate would be one who could say, "I see you want to transition from fossil to alternative fuels. I spent summers working on a farm, I know what the tractors need to do and what current electric vehicle technology can't do. Here's how I think I can help you figure out the solutions."

Lack of proper research is the biggest mistake I see in CVs and interviews these days. Close to it is ego—from both sides. Companies often inflate their jobs the way applicants inflate their resumes. When they have an open job, the HR department may think, "Everybody wants to work for us." Some HR departments also seem to think they're advertising for the next King or Queen of the World. Good candidates have many opportunities and employers should remember that. Whether we're in a tight job market or a wide-open market, companies are looking for that perfect fit for their product or service and existing corporate culture. (They may go looking in different ways in different markets, but they're goal remains the same.) Organisations are looking for the perfect fit for their skill set and candidates are looking for an organisational culture that fits their ethos and lifestyle. At the same time, while some people are insecure about their abilities, some are overconfident and need a good dose of self-awareness about how competitive they actually might be in the job market.

An attractive CV has achievements and I personally like them in specifics. For example, be specific by saying:

"I increased this success by X percentage when the goal was only Y," or "The program I oversaw reduced this problem by Z percentage during that time period."

When I coach MBA students, I help them pull out the specifics that set them apart from other candidates. At London Business School, I coach students who are seeking jobs when they graduate and ask me for advice on their most important calling card, their CV. I might review the CV and start the conversation with, "Okay, I'm looking at what you say you've done and what you're proud of. All this is great, but how is it going to advance the target organization?"

They'll reply, "I did this, this, this, and that."

Then, I'll say, "Right, but what did you achieve from each of those?"

Finally, the conversations becomes useful:

- "I achieved a 12% increase in sales for these products."
- "I achieved a 15% increase in hits to the website among this demographic."
- "I measured our employees for EI/EQ then canvassed staff to ask how they felt they were being treated. Implementing some of their suggestions yielded a 20 % increase in staff job satisfaction."

If you know yourself and know your target company, then you'll know exactly how to present yourself to meet their needs. That is your best path to success. Make it loud and clear on your CV.

INTERVIEWS

FIRST IMPRESSIONS

Some HR professionals believe you can tell within the first minute of an interview if that person has the potential to be hired, or not. To a point, I think that's true. Every interview has a certain "energy"—high or low. Likewise, the interviewer and candidate develop a connection, or they don't. There's also the body language—eye contact, leaning forward, sitting straight, leaning back, how you cross your legs, and more. There's what you say, plus the pace of the dialogue between you and the candidate. Some people just keep talking while others have short, clear answers prepared. Eye contact is important to me. Some people just don't make enough eye contact, revealing an inner lack of interest or insecurity. Others stare. Your subconscious is picking up on cues of how you'll work with the person.

Preparation can also be obvious very quickly. Did you do your homework on the company? Did you do your homework on the person who'll interview you? It's pretty easy to do some homework on Jill Bausch on Google. com or LinkedIn.com and, when people do some homework about me, I notice. A man I interviewed recently said his background was in international trade, then added, "But I know your background is in global health." He'd done his research on me. I immediately thought, "Here's somebody who knows how to prepare."

THE MEETING

Is being interviewed the same thing as submitting a CV? No, but they are similar. They are both building blocks that have to be put together to get the desired outcome. You have total control over what goes into a CV, and no control over how the HR department reacts to it. It's a unidirectional experience for each. An interview is a bi-directional experience for both. They may have a set of standard questions, but might see in you something that takes them totally off-script. Your research probably prepared you to ask specific questions, but something may come up that suggests you take the discussion in a whole new direction. And a line or two about your interests outside of work can be a connection point for an interviewer.

For example, a woman I heard about was an experienced secretary for a mid-level bank executive. She learned of an opening as secretary to three senior executives in another bank in that community. Calling for an interview, she was told the position had closed, they were scheduling no more interviews. The woman, as I did with DFID, got bold and pushed—firmly but gently and politely—for an interview and got one. The interview was with one of the VPs in search of a secretary. He noticed her childhood study of ballet and lamented the fact that his wife and daughter dragged him to sit through *The Nutcracker* every year and how much he hated it.

She responded, "That's because it's the worst ballet ever written." To his shocked expression, she gave him several reasons why she thought so. That led to a 90-minute discussion—of ballet—and she walked out of the interview with a job offer. The VP liked her—her boldness in getting the interview, in criticizing a beloved Christmas tradition, in her ability to defend her opinion with solid reasoning.

Again, I stress, this is the exception to the rule, but I would venture the opinion, based on many years of experience, that it could be a far more common exception if women truly adopted Rachel Platton's "Fight Song" attitude, as quoted in Chapter Three:

Starting right now I'll be strong
I'll play my fight song
And I don't really care if nobody else believes
'Cause I've still got a lot of fight left in me.

In another example, SRI was conducting an initial search for a UN agency that would then do their own interviews and selection. As you can guess, some people are totally comfortable talking about their co-workers' weaknesses or their own, but many are not.

For this search, one applicant and I had the standard discussion on his skill sets, to which he replied, "Here's what I have—an undergraduate degree in psychology, an MBA, 10 years of work experience." All positives.

Then I flipped the straightforward question about weaknesses, asking "What would your team say you need to work on?" He responded, "I've had to work on empathy. I'm really good at high-stress maintenance, but it's hard for me to perceive that other people that are suffering around me. So I really work on that."

We made five recommendations to the agency, and he got a good recommendation from me. He was very forthcoming about what he thinks he did well, what he thinks he can improve. His self-awareness was evident, his desire to improve was evident, and his lack of ego made him compelling. To me, the combination of those qualities says 'high potential'. Looking at the results of his EI/EQ tests, unsurprisingly, corroborated that he was highly interested in self-improvement. People like that are the ones I want to hire or recommend. They have high potential because they are open to learning.

On a closely-related subject, my interviews used to focus on technical competencies, based on the question, "Do they have the skills to do this job?" These questions are still necessary, but I do a lot more in terms of "fit," because I've gotten to know my clients very well. When I ask them what they're looking for in a role, I'm asking them to describe 'the perfect candidate' —what do they look like, walk like, talk like, feel like, when they enter your office? We talk about what a candidate background should be or should not be. Today's hiring authorities seek a really great listener; a person who walks in the room and people immediately pay attention; a person with high EI/EQ; a person who will best fit the organizational culture and help fulfill their mission. Those "soft skills" or "leadership skills" become more and more important as candidates are expected to work with more and more senior government officials, corporate executives, and community leaders.

THE FOLLOW-UP

Part of my job includes keeping in touch with the people we've researched and interviewed and placed in great jobs. As I mentioned before, we have teams all over the world, looking for people to take senior roles with international agencies. In each search, the research team reviews CVs—sometimes hundreds—pares that list down to 10, maybe 20, people to interview for the job. Further interviews and testing may leave us with just five or six final candidates. I usually connect with all of them on LinkedIn, giving me a vast LinkedIn community.

I do try to check in with all of them at least occasionally, with a simple, "How are you doing? How's work going?" Most of them stay in touch with me. They also know the value of establishing relationships. They don't expect to stay in one job forever, so, if you have a headhunter that you know and like, and that you've worked well with before, why wouldn't you keep in touch?

Have I ever placed people in jobs that didn't work out? Of course I have, but technically, no, the client makes the final decision. Still, I recommended that candidate, so part of the responsibility falls to me and SRI Executive. On those rare occasions, we have to work with the employee and the agency to fix it by finding a replacement. I don't think there's any shame in a mistake, only in not fixing it when you need to.

POSITIVE/NEGATIVE FRAMING

As a leader, you should prepare for worst-case scenarios. They happen and they can end your business in a heartbeat. Fortunately, these are rare—earthquakes, fires, floods, terrorist attacks or other circumstances outside your control. That said, you can prepare: Do you have computer backups at a remote location? Do you have cash-on-hand to run the business if income streams are temporarily cut off? Can you keep your people working remotely if your office space becomes unavailable? These things aren't on your daily agenda, but they should always be in the back of your mind.

When I'm getting a briefing for a job search, I put myself in the candidate's place and ask, "Why should I want to work for you?" Obviously, the client frames the response with all the positives they have to offer. As the point of first contact with prospects, I'll relay to them, "Here's why you should be excited about this job."

For example, Gavi, the Vaccine Alliance, is the international alliance providing vaccines to underserved populations, including the vaccines we have for COVID. We were recently retained to find some senior executives for Gavi, and we asked them why candidates would want to work for the alliance. They responded, "Well, if you want to be in the centre of delivering vaccines in the middle of a pandemic, there's no place that you could be except here at Gavi, because we work with populations all over in the world, and not just for pandemic vaccines, but for all the vaccines for children and adults, everywhere. And we saves lives. If you care about this, then you'll want to work here."

That is a powerful statement about their mission and vision and who will fit into the organization. However, I have to create some balance, reminding clients that the best people have other options, because they always do. So, I ask them directly, "What's the downside of working here?"

Concerns could be workload or local political stability. No one could prevent COVID coming, even though medical professionals had been saying for some time that another pandemic was in the cards. COVID changed the priorities for those seeking new roles. Many don't want to come into an office every day, and early research is showing pros and cons of that situation. The lack of connectedness to co-workers is evident, yet many people feel more in control of their lives by going in only two or three days a weeks and working at home for the rest of their work week. If you're looking, consider your views on this before you get to the interview.

Although I believe strongly in the need for all of us to consider Diversity, Equity, and Inclusion (DEI) in everything we do, I will only make one strong point on this here. We have to consider all people for roles and submit balanced, long lists of the best candidates. That means that I have to be looking for any conscious or unconscious bias that may be emanating from clients and candidates. The importance of DEI issues are only going to get more important over time, so whether you're a client looking for a great hire or a person looking for new career opportunities, you'll do yourself a favour by becoming articulate in DEI.

As if in answer to that question, Sri Lanka exploded in mid-2022. As this book was being written, an all-but-dead anti-government protest movement blossomed into a full-blown (but happily non-violent) coup. This came almost on the heels of the war that broke out when Ukraine was attacked by Russia.

These are **global** issues but other potential problems are smaller in scope, though no less difficult to manage. One of them is the movement for DEI, which affects hiring. In trying to reduce this unconscious bias, we sometimes see reverse discrimination.

I can't tell you how many times clients will say, "I want the best person for the job," but they really mean, "I want the best woman for the job." I recently did a major search for an international agency which said they wanted the best person for the job. So, after several months of looking, we found great people— male and female—and submitted the candidates. Then the bomb dropped, "Oh, we're only going to bring the women through."

That's just not being straightforward. I don't mind the client who says, "I have to have a woman, our percentages are too low. I've got to keep balancing out gender." I can deal with just about any limitation on a search, but not wasting people's time, effort, energy, heads, and hearts. That's the height of unprofessional and **disrespectful** behaviour. I have to wonder, if that's the treatment we get during a job search, how are they going to treat people on the job?

As I deal with clients and candidates, I'm expected to deal straight. My reputation, and my company's, is on the line in every search. When I discuss the job with the candidates, it's "Here are the organisation's pros, and here are the challenges you may face." When I present the candidates to the hiring authority, it's the same, "Here are their pros, here are their cons."

Conclusion

Today, CVs need to do two things: Show how you're different from everyone else, and demonstrate your assets, how you can meet their needs. That CV should be customized for each application, based on thorough research of the organization: What are they looking for? What are their needs? How do I fit into their plan and fill their needs?

First impressions are vital to some people, so make a good one. Do some research on the interviewer. Practice potential questions and answers. Video yourself and review it with people who'll give you honest feedback. Be ready for the meeting to go off in some new and unexpected direction. Show your authentic self. If you aren't a fit for them, they aren't a fit for you. Remember that and move on to find your fit.

Understand today's hiring priorities—technical and soft skills, high EI/EQ, an understanding of DEI and how these affect the workplace. Research the company to discern both the positives and negatives of the job, the workplace, the organizational culture, the potential life-disrupting changes you'll have to make. Be aware of the outside forces—medical, political, cultural, linguistic, and others—that could threaten or block your path to success.

There is never a guarantee, but you can always improve the odds vastly with the proper preparation, and packaging yourself as an asset to the organisation.

CHAPTER 10

FIND POWER IN FAILURE

Do not be daunted by the
Enormity of the world's grief.
Do justly, now.
Walk humbly, now.
You are not obligated
To complete the work,
But neither are you free
To abandon it.

—Rabbi Rami Shapiro, *Wisdom of the*
Jewish Sages: A Modern Reading of Pirke Avot[26]

INTRODUCTION — FAILURE

One clear spring morning, I entered my office in the Georgian City of Bath, England. The sign on my office door said, "Chief Executive Officer," and it was my job to manage Futures Group Europe. The world was at the height of the HIV/Aids epidemic and Futures Group worked all over the developing world using government aid money to communicate, teach, and encourage safe sex to stop spreading the AIDS

---

[26] An interpretative rendering of Rabbis Joshua, Yoshe, Shimon, Elazar, and Tarfon's words in Pirkei Avot, 2:11–16 (Ethics/Wisdom of the Fathers), which is itself a commentary on Micah 6:8'.

pandemic that was killing Africa, Asia, and much of the rest of the world.

Some of the bravest people I have met were on street corners in African cities at midnight. People who must sell sex to feed their children. If we could only teach these women ways to make men use condoms then they could live. But many feel, and many are, truly powerless. If only we could teach the drug users not to share needles. If only we could teach the bisexual men to use condoms with each other ... The "if-onlys" never end. But, if not, if they chose to agree to sex without a condom to make the money to feed their kids or buy their drugs or a thousand other things, they were likely to kill themselves and their families.

I had a wonderfully committed staff and, to do this work, we all had to travel frequently to these always vibrant, often destitute, endlessly fascinating places. They were surging with HIV positive people, many who didn't even know or want to know their HIV status. If they knew, they would've had to act by finding condoms and insisting on their use or just wait to die. Many did not want to know their status because they believed something else would kill them sooner, like malaria or typhoid. These are things we rarely thought about in developed countries, although AIDS ravaged those also.

On that day, I had just returned from Kenya a few days before. Almost all the staff traveled, and we casually spoke about trying to avoid getting malaria, deadly and endemic all over Africa—one of the continent's biggest killers. Once the parasites (which live on mosquitos) get inside your bloodstream, they can multiply and overcome your body in days, sometimes hours. It's easy to prevent and to treat, but it's difficult and expensive to get a diagnosis if you're among the poorest and remotest people in the world. Neither I nor my staff wanted to take Larium, the popular anti-malarial drug of that time, because of the drastic side effects. I hadn't taken any on that trip to Kenya.

I casually told the staff, "Just try not to get bitten. If you're near water where mosquitoes congregate, take bug wipes, wipe your ankles, and wear long trousers because they will bite around the ankles, especially at dusk. Spray yourself liberally and frequently."

But I wasn't the leader I should've been. I should've required them to take the anti-malarial drugs to stay alive. It was my duty as CEO. Or, I should've asked them to sign a waiver saying it was their own responsibility if they did not take it.

So, I came in the office, having dropped my kids off at their nearby school in Bath, England, just like any other day. The office was usually quiet at that time of the morning, but I heard rustling in a side office as I walked toward mine. As I sat down at my desk, the Chief Financial Officer, also an early bird, came into my door, ashen-faced.

The evening before, when I left the office, we had discussed the sad turn of events regarding a new staff member, a 36-year-old HIV/Aids specialist, who we had hired from the USA just a few weeks before. She'd taken a trip to Niger, in western Africa, and came back feeling ill. Other staff told me later that she didn't recognise the symptoms she had, and decided to go to emergency at the Bath General Hospital because she felt increasingly unwell. The CFO stood in the doorway and told me that, when he arrived early that morning, the hospital called to tell him she had died. She died of malaria. She hadn't taken the ani-malarial drugs and the parasites flooded into her lungs. Within 24 hours, the parasites induced pulmonary edema—fluid filled her lungs, essentially drowning her to her death in her hospital bed in England.

I heard this news, stunned. It slowly dawned on me that I was responsible. As a board director and company secretary in a UK company, you take on a fiduciary and moral responsibility to protect your staff. I had contravened this entirely and could've been prosecuted for manslaughter, simply by being cavalier about the rules.

When the rest of the staff came to the office, I immediately gathered them all in our picturesque conference room overlooking the beautiful Georgian city, so many miles away from the grit, grime, poverty, and danger of Niger. I told them what happened and that effective immediately, anyone travelling to a high-risk malaria location would take the drugs or choose an option not to travel or sign a waiver of our responsibility for them. They understood and complied, but we all learned the toughest part of tough empathy that day. I hadn't been tough enough and it had cost someone her life. I knew I could not have that on my conscience ever again.

I then had several exceptionally difficult conversations with her family, who understandably blamed me, grilled me about the lack of care I had shown to her. While these debates went on, there were threats to prosecute me, which may have succeeded had they been fulfilled. Her family finally decided not to prosecute, although there were moments when I thought they might. I oversaw the arrangements for having her body sent back to the USA. Just 36 years old, an accomplished doctor with a drive to make the world better than when she came into it, to travel the world and save lives—all those dreams were now behind her forever. Sometimes, tough empathy means being toughest on yourself, and failure is the thing that teaches you the most.

RESILIENT LEADERSHIP

How you cope with failure or other challenging situations defines your resilience.

If you don't cope well when things get tough, you're going to have higher stress levels, lower productivity, and lower all-around well-being. Your level of job satisfaction and general happiness will go down.

As a leader, resilience is vital. People need role models and the leader of the group—parent in the home, teacher in the classroom, supervisor in the office, and so on—sets the tone for the group experience. People need that tone or theme or atmosphere set by the leader. They expect it, because it guides how well they work both individually and collectively.

How do you want to feel and who do you want to feel like? You want to feel like yourself. You want to be authentic, of course, but you also want to feel better. Who appears to feel better about themselves? Who is more confident? Who has more clarity? Who has her life under control? We don't just envy them. We try to emulate them so our lives become more like theirs. It's a natural part of the human psyche. It's exactly what we discussed in Chapter One: "If you don't feel confident, **find a mentor and mirror her**." As a leader, others will be mirroring you.

Leaders, however, must not pretend to be invincible, unaffected by bad news, or "above it all." That's not realistic and the group knows it. As a leader, a measure of detachment is necessary. You and the group members are never completely equals, but blended with a measure of vulnerability. You need to show them your humanity so they feel comfortable enough around you to share their concerns. If you present yourself as aloof and unfeeling, they won't share when you need them to share. They won't trust you.

As with everything else, it is balance. Strength and resilience gives the leader power to convincingly say, "We can get through this. We'll make it happen. We're stronger together." Because, if the leader crumbles in a challenge, how are the group members going to get through it? On the other side of the coin, when times get tough, group members may need a little hand-holding, extra encouragement, understanding. A leader who projects the "Shut up and soldier on!" attitude is more likely to lose employees when they are needed most.

So, what has to happen when disaster strikes? Major disasters—life and death scenarios—or small disasters—the inevitable delays and mistakes we can never eliminate—the process is the same, only the scale and the timetable changes.

Resilience is the ability to spring back, to go to Plan B, to cover for each other, to suffer through bad times and keep going. Don't feel hesitant about saying, for example, "Okay, J is down with a serious flu, will be out a week. We can't wait for her to get back to finish this project. That throws us all for six, but okay. Now, everybody go to your desks, wallow in self-pity for half an hour, because we'll be putting in some major overtime to get the job done. Then look at the To-Do list, meet me in the conference room, and tell me who can cover for what J was going to do. I'm running out to get J a get-well-soon card and some flowers. I will see you in one hour. We will then figure it out and make it happen."

If it's a real (i.e., life-altering) tragedy, things will take longer, obviously. Give them and yourself the time and space everyone needs, but keep in the back of your mind, "and then I need to reorder my world to the new normal, get back into my world (my new world, with a new understanding and a new set of rules), and feel like I can do all that again." Then do just that.

TOUGH TIMES DEMAND TOUGH MINDS—AND STOOL LEGS

I'd like to say that life-altering tragedies are rare, and maybe they are, but I think we're living in particularly turbulent times. Previous generations had world wars and a global depression, we have the war on terror and COVID, to name just a couple. They, at least, had a very public enemy—you knew where the threat originated. Today's threats are stealthy. You really can't predict where the next disaster may arise.

In Chapter Five, I mentioned my boss at Marriott Hotels, who died in the terrorist attack over Lockerbie, Scotland. That was a pivotal moment for me. I could've had a completely different life because of that incident. I could've been worried all the time. You read about people who go through devastating trauma and that's how they react. They choose to live a closeted life, protected (they think) from fear of the outside world because they (as much as possible) refuse to interact with the world. There are certainly people still suffering from that attitude now, after we've essentially come through the pandemic. Things are opening up all over the world. Most places are trying hard to get back to "business as usual," but not the people who can't come back from serious trauma. They've become so used to holding themselves in, they're afraid to let go.

"A place for everything and everything in its place," they used to say. Well, suppose that, suddenly, you feel like the "place for everything" has moved, and you're not sure where it's gone. I certainly feel that, at times. When I do, I try to make my world smaller, to remember what's working. I ask myself, "What can you do now?" "What's working now that you can hold on to?"

My brother, Dan—a very accomplished specialist in hemorrhagic fevers, particularly Ebola—lives in Geneva, Switzerland. He's fond of the "three-legged stool" theory, which we believe applies to every person on the planet. This is our "stool leg" analogy for life: One stool leg is your health and wellbeing; another leg is what you do to feel worthwhile—paid employment or volunteer work; maybe this is toiling in the fields, maybe this is running an international organization, maybe this is volunteering your time at a charity; the final leg is your relationships—spouse, partner, family, friends, kids, other associates, the people who are meaningful in your life. If things are not going easily with one leg, you'll have one leg off the ground. The stool can still balance fairly easily with two, but it requires constant attention not to topple over. If two legs are off the ground, it's generally all you can do to keep the stool upright. And sometimes you'll be feeling that all three stool legs are in the air. At those times its very challenging to muster the energy and bravery to deal with all three getting grounded again.

Dan and I are very close. We talk about everything. He might start a phone call with, "How are your stool legs doing?" I might respond, "Okay, right now: My relationships with my partner and children are firm, just the usual family issues. My professional life is very solid— I'm busy, well-paid, I like what I do and feeling lucky doing it. I make the time to give away time to some that need it. My health is good, too—I'm not as social as I was before the pandemic, but that's okay. Overall,

197

I feel like all the legs are down and firm." Sometimes, one of our stool legs is off the ground, but Dan and I talk each other through it. Sometimes in life, we both have had all three off the ground, and that's when you need to give yourself some time and grace to work through it.

A conversation like that is, actually, a "More of/Less of" exercise. It's a way to say, "Where have I got a handle on things? What do I need to work and focus on?"

Priorities

Each of the stool legs should has equal priority and, in a perfect world, they would, all the time. In the real world, each must take its turn. One way to set priorities is to say, "What can I make happen right now and what can't I?"

This became clear to me a few years ago. I went into the hospital for minor surgery and was infected with MRSA (methicillin-resistant staphylococcus aureus, if you care for details). It's one of the risks of being in a hospital, and I ended up spending two months in two different hospitals. Frankly, they didn't know if I was going to live. I was 48.

There I was, IVs dripping into my arm day and night for nine weeks, and there wasn't one thing I could do to change that. After my discharge, I still didn't have energy—couldn't even walk up the stairs to my bedroom. Fortunately, I found help and I got stronger, over time. All I could do was wait for my body to heal itself. But, while I was doing that, I thought, "Well, I can get my work in order." My brain was fully functional, even though my body wasn't. So, I worked on what needed attention and creativity—new clients and old friends. My family was very supportive and keeping my mind active prevented massive boredom and the stress that would've accompanied it. I had two legs solidly on the ground which made having that one shaky leg something I could handle.

It reminded me of the famous principle used by Alcoholics Anonymous:

> God grant me the
> Serenity to accept the things I cannot change, the
> Courage to change the things I can, and the
> Wisdom to know the difference.

That last line, I think, is the key—the wisdom to know what you can do, what you can have an effect upon and what you have to wait for. If you let the things that you can't change control you, they'll constantly draw you down and life's going to be a tough road.

THE BENEFITS

> Failure should be our teacher, not our undertaker. Failure is delay, not defeat. It is a temporary detour, not a dead end. Failure is something we can avoid only by saying nothing, doing nothing, and being nothing.[27]

---

[27] Denis Waitley, *Psychology of Winning: Ten Qualities of a Total Winner*. London: Penguin Publishing Group, 1986.

Failure has benefits. It provides lessons that are more in the soft skills than the technical, but these are infinitely valuable in your toolbox. Two examples:

HUMILITY

When my co-worker died, I learned to be tougher. Most rules exist for a purpose and I ignored that purpose. I'm now tougher and less cavalier. The greater lesson, though, was humility. Look at any leadership study and you'll probably find that people who practice tough empathy are humble. Humans' natural state becomes encased in one of ego, a selfishness tied to our survival instinct. With few exceptions (narcissists, psychopaths, sociopaths), humans have learned that cooperative measures enhance survival probabilities. Still, our egotistical tendencies can get away from us—thinking we are always right, thinking our way is always the best way, and such.

Failure, through unplanned or deliberate incidents of tough empathy, humbles us. It proves we are not as smart as we think we are and helps us reign in those "law of the jungle" tendencies. When we recognize those failures for what they are—learning opportunities—we can extend that learning to others via mentoring and coaching. I believe those who really achieve things of significance must have a great measure of humility because they know they're just human.

COMPASSION

Compassion can be another lesson from failure. Once you feel failure, you can have compassion, or empathy, for the failures of others. Remember, every person you cross in the street, every person you see or speak to has their own difficulties. They have work to do on themselves, challenges to bear. Be compassionate. Be kind. Be nice. But don't be weak.

PRACTICAL FACTORS – LET'S PLAY A GAME

Take the following quiz:

WHO? After being cut from his high school basketball team, he went home, locked himself in his room, and cried.

Michael Jordan—6-time time National Basketball Association Champion, 5-time NBA Most Valuable Player, 4-time NBA All-Star Player.

He said, "I can accept failure, but I can't accept not trying."

WHO? He wasn't able to speak until he was four years old and was told by teachers that he would never amount to much.

Albert Einstein—world renowned physicist and Nobel Laureate, author of the famous $e=mc^2$.

He said, "A person who has never made a mistake has never tried anything new."

WHO? She was demoted from her job as a news anchor and was told she "was not fit for television."

Oprah Winfrey—host of a multi-award-winning talk show, voted one of the "Most Influential Women in the World" by numerous media, winner of the Golden Global Award for Lifetime Achievement, and the US Presidential Medal of Freedom.

She said, "Failure is another stepping-stone to greatness."

WHO? After almost 21 years of continuous service in the British Cabinet, he was dismissed from all posts and so ostracized that no one thought he'd ever be invited back into the halls of power.

Winston Churchill—Prime Minister of the UK during World War II, the man most responsible for the defeat of world domination by the Nazis.

He said, "Never give in—never, never, never, never, in nothing great or small, large or petty, never give in except to convictions of honour and good sense."

WHO? At 30 years old, he was left devastated and depressed after being unceremoniously removed from the company he founded.

Steve Jobs—founder of Apple, Inc., first public company in the USA to be valued at $1 trillion; he changed the way the world communicates.

He said, "Have the courage to follow your heart and your intuition. Time is limited—don't waste your life living someone else's."

WHO? They were rejected by Decca Records, who said they did not like their sound and they had no future in show business.

The Beatles—Grammy and Academy Award® winning musicians, the most influential group in musical history.

They said, "There's nowhere you can be that isn't where you're meant to be..."

WHO? His fiancé died, he failed in business, had a nervous breakdown, and was defeated in eight elections.

Abraham Lincoln—16th President of the United States, globally-recognised as one of the greatest leaders of all time.

He said, "Always bear in mind that your own resolution to succeed, is more important than any other one thing."

Failure plus resilience plus reflection plus realignment can equal success, power, and a sublime sense of achievement while allowing you to maintain your authentic self.

Resilience derives from the Latin *resili*, meaning "to spring back." What does it mean to be resilient?

- Being open to learning and self-growth, intellectually and emotionally.

- Being able to take risks with the confidence that whatever the outcome, you have the power to deal with it.
- Being able to manage well through a setback; to get back on the proverbial horse.

Ask yourself "Am I resilient?" Look for these signs in yourself demonstrating a lack of resilience:

- Are you a presenter with something meaningful to say who avoids speaking opportunities?
- Are you a leader who procrastinates decisions?
- Do you exhibit strong negative emotions when positive energy and thought are needed?
- Do you show volatile or inconsistent behaviour towards others?
- Do you tend to fixate on one solution only, while just giving lip service to others?
- Do you avoid social situations which could benefit you or those who work for you?

Look at the following list of characteristics. Which traits do you recognise in yourself?

Person A

Has higher levels of serotonin, above average resilience, and variants of genes linked to a natural ability for emotional intelligence. Common traits of a highly emotionally intelligent person:

- Naturally optimistic, despite problems
- Capable of restoring equilibrium and resetting their stress levels after failure

- Able to access their cognitive powers and EQ traits easily
- Able to examine emotional tone created in the aftermath of a set back and react in support of others, rather than punitively
- Has the energy and desire to move forward despite failure

PERSON B

Has gene variants which result in higher level of adrenaline, but lower ability to remain functional in stressful situations, greater volatility of emotional and intellectual responses, less flexible to adapt to changes in circumstances. Common traits of a lower emotionally intelligent person:

- Overwhelmed by stress of events which may seem negative
- Creates further negative narratives which do not allow them to see a future or past failure
- Finds it difficult to imagine they can do anything other than what they have ordinarily done, but may give lip service to change

CREATING RESILIENCE IN YOURSELF

Each of us needs to understand our own level of resilience:

- Can you work with colleagues well at a level beyond which you would not go yourself?
- Are you familiar with your own areas of vulnerability?

- Do you know what sparks your own anxiety, pushes your own tolerance limits? What are your habitual responses?

We've already discussed feedback and noted that "Performance measured is performance improved." So, consider these questions for a private, personal evaluation:

- Can you hold the mirror up to your own thought processes and behaviors?
- Can you reframe narratives from negatives to positives and find silver linings?
- Do you listen or just hear? How would you know if you're really listening? (Be specific.)
- Are your solutions focused? How would you know? (Be specific.)
- Do you diffuse stress or create it? How? (Be specific.)

EXERCISES

Consider an unsatisfactory professional situation that you wish you could rewind and replay.

- How would you replay that situation?
- Could you have been more resilient? How? (Be specific.)
- How might resilience have affected the outcome, the sense of achievement, the sense of well-being?

Consider six common habits that contribute to your sense of failure. Ask yourself, do I:

1. Dither, dither, dither, plan, plan, plan.

   Instead: Decide early—not impulsively, but early. If you fail, fail fast, recoup, stay flexible.

   Make decisions earlier to create options and build flexibility. Postponing decisions in the attempt to optimize your results can waste your resources in other ways and reduce your options. Fear of making the wrong decision (or of failure) creates higher risk of failure by the delay.

2. Fight the fight, never let someone get the better of you.

   Instead: Pick the right battles, at the right time, with the right people. Let the others go.

   Stand up for yourself and be firm, but keep your ego in check. Big egos get in the way of good ideas.

   Make prudent decisions based on your present situation and capabilities and your best guess as to future resources and prospects, rather than fighting every battle that comes your way. Learn to walk away when victory comes at too high a price.

3. Over-promise, over-sell, under-deliver.

   Instead: Realistically-promise, over-deliver.

   When in doubt, do less. When you pace yourself properly, you're more efficient, more productive, more in control, and you reduce your contribution to the normal stress of the situation, creating an environment of well-being and power.

4. Be stubborn in the face of failure.

   Instead: Be determined in the face of disbelief.

   Flexibility is a virtue, not a weakness; error is inevitable, so accept being wrong and make more mistakes to learn better and faster. Good ideas need determination despite setbacks.

5. "I/they know more than anyone else…"

   Instead: If you think you (or the boss) are the smartest person in the room, you're creating stress, not well-being. Even if you are the smartest person in the room, you are probably not also the wisest, the most experienced, the most talented, the most skilled, the nicest, the most fun, the most just-about-anything-else. Do what you do best, let others shine in their areas.

   Teams bring everyone along. Egos put others in the shadows. If you do that, you're stopping your idea from working best because you're sucking the motivation from the people who can make the idea work to its fullest.

   If you think you're always right, (A) you're not; (B) you've picked the wrong co-workers. Hire and work with people smarter or more talented than you in some way. Listen to them. Look for people who challenge your ideas. Take the blame for failures, give away the credit for successes, and, once in a while, take one for the team. Give your ego the week off.

6. Meet to discuss.

   Instead: Meet to decide.

   Meetings to disseminate information are the biggest timewaster in almost all organizations. In meetings, structure an agenda that leads to decisions being made on the spot whenever possible. Assign responsibilities in that meeting, not later. Find other means of disseminating information.

Now, consider again that professional situation. We will not, today, consider how it went wrong or how to fix what went wrong. We are focused on how failure affects you. To repeat:

**Failure + Resilience + Reflection + Realignment =
Power & Achievement.**

So, what are you going to do about **you**? Mitigate the effects of failure in four steps:

1. Break the bad news yourself.

   If you've made a mistake, don't hope that no one will notice. They will. When someone else points out your failure, that one failure is compounded. By staying quiet, others will attribute this to either cowardice or ignorance. Have the emotional intelligence to speak up. Humans are fallible, let yourself be human. (It's really not as bad as some people say it is.)
2. Always offer an explanation, never make an excuse.

Owning your mistakes will always gain you great *face*. It demonstrates confidence, accountability, and integrity. Just be sure to stick to the facts. "We lost the account because I missed the deadline," is a reason. "We lost the account because I wasn't sure what to put in the presentation," is an excuse, and a powerless position.

3. Have a plan to correct it, for now.

   Owning up to a mistake is one thing, but you can't end it there. Life goes on. It is critical to offer your own solutions. Tell your colleagues the specific steps that you've already taken to get things back on track, and what you plan to do. Ask for their input.

4. Have a plan to prevent it in the future.

   Develop preventative measures or protocols so you'll avoid repetition of that error. Again, include input from co-workers where appropriate. Reassure people that the problem was temporary and a one-off. Unburden yourself of past mistakes so you're free to make new mistakes! (And learn from them!)

CONCLUSION

Failure is inevitable and many of history's most successful people failed more often than they succeeded.

It is neither a sin nor a disgrace to fail, it is both a sin and a disgrace to let a past failure define your future.

Resilience means experiencing "The slings and arrows of outrageous fortune"[28] and maintaining the ability to spring back, keep your group together, cover for each other, suffer through bad times, and get the job done. We talk a great deal about resilience in leaders but, of course, the same holds true for every member of the group because, if one fails, all might fail.

The situation in the modern world is changing, quickly and unpredictably, maybe more so than at any other period in history. How can you feel you have everything in its place when you feel that the places where things belong keep moving in new and strange directions? When life seems completely out of control, it isn't. Some things are still working. Focus on what's working. Ask yourself, "What can I do now?" "What can I hold on to?" Build from there.

---

[28] William Shakespeare, *The Tragedy of Hamlet, Prince of Denmark*, Act III, Scene 1, Line 1751.

CHAPTER 11
TURBULENT TIMES

Come with me to a quiet place,
Where sun and breeze and sand erase
Troubles, conflict, senseless chatter
Come with me to find what matters
most—
Holding you,
I find my heaven close.

—Hallmark

INTRODUCTION — HANNAH

We named her Hannah. Now, she's a woman that had I longed to be when I was younger, but I couldn't find her in me back then. Hannah came home one day to her middle-class house in a happy, middle-class life in Bath, England, and said her knees hurt. She was 11. I remembered rolling my eyes upward, while doing all the things mothers do simultaneously, like looking after other kids, fixing dinner, wondering when a glass of wine would appear, and wondering when I could get some of my own time to catch up on my own work.

I told Hannah with a tinge of exasperation, "Well you've probably fallen down in sports class, or in gym, and didn't you stumble on the stairs last week?" Hannah replied, "Well, yes, but it still hurts to walk Mummy."

Hannah has long, thick, shiny, red-auburn hair—the kind that people stop on the street to admire. On that day years ago, she had that wonderful hair on the outside and an old, wise, knowing soul on the inside. A soul that never complained though you knew she had known suffering and had learned to endure it over days and months—perhaps centuries.

After that first day, Hannah came home day after day, and week after week, saying her knees hurt more, her wrists hurt, most of her joints hurt. Finally, I started to listen, but just a bit. I took her to a physiotherapist out of doubt and frustration. The physio told me, "She's just self-absorbed and making this up for attention. I can find nothing wrong with her. She just needs to grow up." Hannah was still just 11.

The next week, I took Hannah and her brother on a trip to Disney World in Florida. But after the 9-hour flight, Hannah tried to walk off the plane and couldn't. Her joints wouldn't bend, wouldn't let her to stand up and walk. She was a prisoner. We found an airport wheelchair and I started to doubt all the doubts I had, and I started to really listen.

Hannah's father, still in the UK, also had pains in his joints, which had started a few weeks before we left. In Florida, we spent the first night in a hotel and, as we went to bed, Hannah saw a Waffle House across the street. She was excited to go there the next morning. But when we woke up early to cross the road for waffles, Hannah couldn't walk without her brother and me on each arm to support her.

We finally made it the short distance to the Waffle House, slid into a red shiny booth, ate breakfast, and laughed. After that, Hannah slept the whole day. No Disney World for us just yet. The next day Hannah woke up excited again, but immobile. She could not move. She fell back into bed, exhausted. When I woke her later to get up and go, because I was still in denial, still wanting to believe it was jet lag or travel fatigue and she would be back to normal the next day. She always wanted to go to Disney World so, the following morning, she dragged herself from the bed to go, accepted a wheelchair because she didn't have the energy or mobility to walk to the rides she rode. She hummed, "It's a Small, Small, World."

Smiling effusively through the Small World ride, she took pics with Disney characters, but could hardly move. She even joked "that 'wheelchair gig' was pretty good because it put us all at the front of the line."

I finally woke up; Hannah was seriously ill. Three days later, we flew back to England. Before we flew to Florida, she'd gone with her father to the doctor and told him that she too, had pains in her joints. In fact, both had the same symptoms. The doctor took blood samples from Hannah and her father and, on our return, the results had come back. Her father had been told he had very temporary rheumatoid arthritis symptoms, which were rare but would go away eventually.

Hannah wasn't so lucky, she had polyarticular juvenile arthritis, a devastating disease that eats away at the joints in the body. The fluid in her joints, for reasons not entirely known, attack the joints, breaking them down, causing enormous pain and disability. It's a cruel disease that for many results ends in astonishing disability. It's also a life sentence, without reprieve, except for the wonderful in-roads science is now making in drugs to combat it. If you can get the drugs.

Hannah spent much of the next year in Bristol Temple Meads hospital in Bristol, England, enduring endless drug infusions and joint treatment. I sat by her side every minute I could, going back and forth to my job as CEO at Futures Group Europe in Bath, trying to look after my staff, manage the business, care for her younger brother, and thoroughly feeling that he was not getting the attention and care a 9-year-old kid should have. Her dad, while loving, was not very engaged, and his conflict-adverse personality was a principal reason we'd divorced a few years earlier. He lived 100 miles away and, because he did not handle stress very well, stayed away most of the time. I tried to do what all parents try to do—just keep everything together—while feeling I wasn't doing a great job at any of the important jobs that life had handed me. All my stool legs were flying sky high.

One day, I was sitting with Hannah in the hospital. She had endless drip needles inserted into her which allowed the miracle drugs access to her joints. But that day, I could see the sadness darkening her face, while she said nothing. That moment scared me more than anything because I knew in my heart that state of mind is everything. I turned to the nurse, and said, "She's just 12, she needs an hour of normal life. Please."

That nurse, about my age, probably with kids of her own, gave me a knowing look. She drew the curtains round Hannah's bed; we were out of sight of the rest of the ward. That blessed nurse then unhooked the tubes inserted in Hannah's arms, leaving the needles in, but taping them over to stay clean. She covered up Hannah's drip sites and helped her put a sweatshirt over them. She gave Hannah a wink and said, "You're 12—go for two hours, be free, walk, and breathe. Maybe you'll buy something nice to eat, and just be with your Mum."

That nurse sprung us, just for two hours, but those two hours were the best hours of Hannah's life up to that moment, and the best hours of mine. And that nurse was a saviour with her act of compassion and flexibility.

TURBULENT TIMES

I've used that term or idea before, discussing the things in the world that affect our lives—the external turbulence over which we have no control—an illness or accident, natural disasters, other people's bad behaviour, and more. For the final part of our discussion, let's consider the internal turbulences over which we have control. I should say that my daughter's situation was, as many are, a combination. Even if we have no control over the events, we always have control over how we react to and deal with the event.

Hannah is now a successful executive in New York, with many surgeries behind her and probably many more to come. Her hands have been rebuilt more than once; she has bars on her bones where her wrists used to be. But it doesn't stop her from laughing and crying and toasting a great life. She has that same old soul that never complains. She just fixes what is broken.

Hannah is the bravest woman I know.

As I was writing this book, a work situation arose for me that, I think, exemplifies how these situations should be handled:

To put it simply, for the first time in a long time, I felt like I was working way too much—like a gerbil on a wheel. I'd been getting up and having calls from eight in the morning to eight at night, with five minutes in between calls, if I was lucky. I was doing a large number of psychometrics analyses—maybe 40, maybe 50—in a very short time. These require analysis and feedback to everybody who does one, and many senior headhunting roles now require them.

So, I said to my partner, "This is not what I envisaged. I don't want to be a workaholic, even though it's generating a good income." He's not as affected by overwork as I am, because he's a banker and he's always been on call. He has even worked on many a Christmas Day. But I need more work-life balance. I decided over a weekend that change was needed to get my balance back. He really doesn't want to be financially responsible for another person (he's been there), nor do I want someone else responsible for me. He's a good soul, though. He said, "Of course I'll look after you if something happens, but you have a job to do, too." He was right—I love my work, principally because it has real value for the world, and I don't want to give that up.

However, too much of a good thing ...

The overwork was having a bad effect on me, making me feel like life was passing by and I might be missing other good parts of life. I don't have **FOMO**—Fear Of Missing Out. I don't feel a need to go out every night, never have. But there are things in life other than your job and I wanted to do what was good for me and those I loved. There were things I just didn't want to miss.

So, what to do about the overworking? I decided, "I'll modulate it where I can and hopefully clients will modulate it where they can and we'll meet where it works for all of us." I sat down for a crucial conversation with myself: I thought, "Okay, what can I delegate? What can I rebalance in my work life? What can go from the To-Do list the Not-To-Do list?"

I went through all the things that people wanted me to do every day—not an exaggeration, every day, someone was asking me to do something more. After careful analysis, I decided I would say no to some additional big-ticket work.

At SRI's headquarters in Dublin, Ireland, contracts were streaming in for major searches and they pulled me into a lot of proposals. SRI would call me and say, "Okay, we want you to lead the search for this position," and I agreed about 99 percent of the time.

Well, obviously, it wouldn't be professional or ethical for me to simply leave them in the lurch by just saying no to everything. Instead, I sent a note to SRI's CEO saying, "Seamus, can I have a chat with you?" Of course, he said yes immediately, and we chatted. To summarize:

I started with "I feel like I'm a gerbil in a wheel at the moment, and for the last few months. I'm ever grateful for the work ... (I'm a consultant, not an employee, so, more work means more pay) ... and we've worked together for nine years. I love working with you. I love the company. I love what we do. I love the mission. My heart's in it, but I can't balance my life as things now stand. And I don't want to. I'll keep doing the psychometrics, because I can't delegate those and I love doing those. (You have to be certified to do those and he didn't have someone to replace me at that time.) I'll keep doing the coaching because I can't delegate that, ... but please don't give me any new roles to take on for a month."

He said, "I completely understand. But I do need to know whether you're in for the next two or three years. This is not the beginning of you going away, is it?"

I assured him it was not.

He then said, "What if we get a really senior, huge role in the global health world? What if we get retained for that?" He knows that's my background and where my heart is.

I told him, "For that, I'll make an exception." However, I also told him I felt the need to get working on this book. I had a message I needed to share through the book. Once it was written, I also had to promote the book. I framed that as having a cake and not eating it— spending the time, the effort and emotional energy on the book, but then not seeing it read by women who need it because I wasn't doing anything to actively promote it. I wanted to get these messages out there.

He understood that, too.

So, it was agreed: He wouldn't give me new search work for the next month. Seamus is a great boss with super high EQ and he knew that my stool legs were flying high or I wouldn't have asked for a reprieve.

This was, at that moment, some minor turbulence, but one that could've easily grown into a major upheaval had he not understood and been patient. To prevent that, I set expectations for my work. I set boundaries with my Not-To-Do list. He comprehended instantly that he had a crucial conversation on his hands and went to Level 3 listening. He listened, agreed, but asked for a Plan B, if he needed one. We recognized a pivotal moment and we pivoted to a new direction that met both our needs.

And we stuck to it. Rebalance achieved!

(And by the way, that huge global health role came in, and I did accept leading it, but managed my balancing efforts around it.)

LESSONS LEARNED

LOSS OF CONTROL

I think in almost every problem in anyone's life—be it personal, professional, any other arena—if you feel like you don't have any control, the situation is automatically worse for you. So, when I sat down and thought this all through, I concluded, "You can say no, and you can do it in a kind way. You can give Seamus a heads up. You can say, 'I'd love to, but I'm resourced to the hilt right now.'" That was taking control back in a non-aggressive, non-confrontational way.

Another part of the problem, I think, was the feeling that, since we can be out and about again, without pandemic fears, people are getting back into the habit of getting out. I didn't want to be in a position that I had to say, "I'm working all the time, I couldn't go out and do anything anyway." That's unbalanced and self-limiting.

During this time, I went to a Bob Marley exhibition, but I had to block that time on my calendar a month and a half prior. Now, I can be more spontaneous. Feeling like I'm in control again, I feel that, if I have something I'm interested in doing, I can go do it without deserting others who depend on me.

Likewise, instead of telling someone I won't have 10 minutes to talk on the phone with them for the next two weeks, I can set work aside. Part of my feeling of self-worth is tied to being available to people who need me. Not every person, not all the time, but for family, friends, co-workers and others in my inner circles, feeling that I couldn't give them even 15 minutes in a two-week period was not acceptable.

I should add that it felt better immediately. Even the day after my chat with Seamus, I wasn't thinking, "Ah, how do I say no to the next thing somebody asks me to do?" I'd said it, the decision was made.

Having set some new boundaries, setting others also became easier. While the book was in the publishing pipeline, we did some pre-publication advertising, and I got a request from a big consulting company, "Will you come and talk to my management group, with offices all over Europe, about the important messages in this book?" I was able to say, "Sure." As we talked it through, I sent the contact the chapter titles and said, "Look, can we make it easier for me by doing this as an interview rather than a speech? You can have a senior person in the company ask me questions after I do a short intro. I don't want to write out a speech, I'm more comfortable with you folks just asking whatever you want to ask." They immediately agreed and it worked much better in two-way communication, with the audience also asking questions, than a one-way speech would have been anyway. They got what they needed, I saved some time and it was a great success. Lateral thinking at work!

Autonomy

Working is important because it creates self-reliance, which builds self-esteem, security, and more. But there are some aspects of work that are a double-edged sword. Many people are excited to get back to the office, at least part time, after the pandemic. They like the separation of home and work lives, they thrive on the synergy of the group experience, and for other reasons. Many others don't want to go back to the office five days a week or work from eight to six. These people value autonomy and flexibility over those other factors. For myself, the autonomy has always been my number one priority. More than money, more than anything else, I want maximum control over my situation, to be able to do it when I want to do it. I've never missed a deadline and I don't intend to. As long as I get the work done on time and within the budget, the rest, I feel, should be up to me. There was no space for autonomy when I was working 12 to 14 hours a day.

It's a benefit that people are learning to value their own time, and they're finding time at home to do the work plus other things, like write that book they've been thinking about for years. Self-improvement book sales are through the roof post-pandemic, as many of you already know. People are starting to think, "Okay, what is important to me in my life?" I mean, after we dealt with the panic of the last two years—when we thought half the world might give up the ghost and still could—now we're on the verge of another European war. We are all reevaluating our life priorities, roles and values. Whoever thought that would happen? We are so powerless to control so many things, people are wanting to take control of what they can control and they're thinking about their legacy. They're asking: "So, how do I want to spend the time I have? What will I leave behind?"

As we go back to work, your own office situation might give you the space to do that, but it might not. That's why we're seeing the **Great Resignation**, which I prefer to call the **Great Re-Evaluation**. That's one reason we have the self-help genre screaming through the roof, because we've all had more time at home to think about: "Is what I'm doing meaningful? Do I know what's meaningful for me?"

We're seeking a new or better purpose in life. And we're asking what tools can I use to help me figure out what my purpose is? No one wants to live a life they think lacks any purpose, any point, any value in the grand scheme of things.

All this follows from increased autonomy.

COACHING

No one is entirely autonomous, unless you live alone in a cabin in the woods. A community is an interactive situation. It has to be collaborative to operate well. Within that community, every person knows more than you do, about one subject or another. And you know more than others. You have your own bank of knowledge. Everyone does. Likewise, within that community, every person knows less than you do, about one subject or another. To create the best-case scenario, we need to get the right people doing their best at what they do best. Being clear about what your banks of knowledge hold is important in the reassessment process.

For any of you to do your best, coaching is essential. Before he became a science fiction writer, Gene Roddenberry was a Los Angeles, California, police officer, and he wrote some articles for the department magazine. In one article, he proposed seven hallmarks of a profession, including:

- A duty to continually work to improve skills by all means available and to freely communicate professional information gained...
- A duty to give constant attention to the improvement of self-discipline, recognizing that the individual must be the master of himself to be the servant of others.[29]

The benefits of coaching cannot be overstated. They go far beyond just the self-improvement Roddenberry suggests. Coaching gives someone the ability to figure out for themselves the answers to the questions they have and how to best manage the problems they face. So, I've been coached and I became a certified coach as well. What many people tend to want to do is offer you solutions to fix things. Most of us are not seeking that, and benefit more by being encouraged to think laterally about our own issues so that we can seek, find, and evaluate alternatives to improve our situation. That's what coaching does.

---

[29] Eugene Wesley "Gene" Roddenberry, in *The Beat*, September 1952, quoted in David Alexander, *Star Trek Creator: The Authorized Biography of Gene Roddenberry*. London: Penguin Publishing Group, 1994.

If you say, "I really don't like the way my project's going," many people will reply, "Why don't you do this? Why don't you do that? Why don't you try what I did when this happened to me?"

This isn't coaching. Coaching requires thought provoking questions, not suggested answers. Questions like:

- Well, could you think of anything differently?
- What would happen if you tried to think about this situation in that different way?
- Who would be in your way if you tried to say yes or no to something?
- What would open up for you if you reframed this situation differently in your thinking about it?

In coaching we start with the premise that everybody has more inside them than they realise. Then, when they figure it out themselves and start saying things like, "Maybe I could try this, this, and this," you leave them for a time to try this, this and this. Hopefully, they'll find the answers were already inside them and they'll come back and say, "Yeah, I don't know what was holding me back from doing that," or "I simply hadn't thought of it in that way." Each success will increase their self-esteem because they've worked it out themselves. I like to think of coaching as taking a lump of clay and telling others to mould a pot, instead of showing them a specific pot and telling them to replicate it. They then figure what kind of pot it should be.

I like the words **power** and **confidence**. I think the term "empowering" has been overused, but I do like the idea of confidence and power going together, because when you get confidence, you have more power. That's what some women seem to be lacking. With a good coach, they realize they have the power. It doesn't have to be aggressive or hard, it can, in fact, be very soft, very gentle—persuasive instead of forceful power—but they have it and, when they understand they have it, they can fix most anything.

A great example comes from a study I heard about: In a certain nursing home, they gave participating residents a plant. Half the residents watered it themselves and half were told the nurses would water it. There was a noticeably greater improvement of mood among those residents who watered their own plants.

Instill in someone the ability to do for themselves and, even though all you did was just give them a nudge in the right way, you did enough. The rest they could do for themselves.

I can't think of a better gift to give other people.

ANXIETY

As I often say to my partner, Austin, in the years we've been together, "There's a lot of ∫#!+ going down"—pandemics, militarism, political upheaval, environmental challenges, rampant inflation, war, civil unrest, the repeal of Roe v. Wade—you name it! You don't know what's going to blow up next. You feel the world is out of control, so you must be also. **If it isn't getting better, and it's easy to think it won't, why bother?** Digesting these macro world issues each day can be difficult. Call it anxiety or suffering (I think they're pretty much two sides of the same coin), they rob you of **clarity of thinking.**

Realising this and moderating how much of the outside craziness you take in may be a good tool in your own personal toolbox. Consider how much you need and want. While **hope** is not a strategy, nor is wishful thinking, I think hope and gratitude are essential for peaceful living and productive thinking. Science shows that those who actively practice gratitude either by writing down two or three things they are grateful for each day or even making that list in their head, have better mental health, higher levels of contentment and longer lives.

A study from University of California at Berkeley shows that active gratitude can improve stress levels, feelings of happiness, and overall mental health.[30] So put gratitude in your toolbox every day!

While the world is swirling with troubling issues you can't control, you can certainly control your gratitude list.

Some of us cope with anxieties by ignoring them. But like mold or mice in the walls, they don't go away, they just get worse. Each of us must find the specific coping mechanisms that work best for us. A few suggestions:

- Do something for somebody else. It doesn't have to be a big thing; even small things can be life-changing: Give a bit of money to a charity.

---

[30] https://greatergood.berkeley.edu/article/item/how_gratitude_changes_you_and_your_brain

Volunteer for a few hours at the senior center, care facility, food bank. Write a letter to a friend and just ask them how they're doing. When was the last time you received something like that? Plant a tree. Give up your seat on a crowded bus. Compliment a co-worker. Sign an organ donor card. Give some books to a school.

- Think about what *is* working. Almost everybody can focus, at any time, on one aspect of their lives that is working. You may want to take pen to paper and make a list. I find the act of writing it out is a cathartic act that gets it out of my head and in front of my eyes, even though I'm not really a good journal-keeper. Some people journal every morning or evening. I don't, but when I think about what's working, I want to see it in front of me. My son once gave me a little book entitled, *My Gratitude List*. So, when feel overwhelmed, I can write 10 things in this digest in half a minute or less.

- Create something to look forward to. Even if it's small and simple, such as, "I look forward to the end of the day and having a glass of wine," or "I look forward to a chocolate chip biscuit with breakfast." It could also be something big, such as, "I look forward to a holiday planned with my boyfriend," or "I look forward to a big, old-fashioned, family dinner." Anything—put a dinner date in the diary, send a girlfriend a text saying, "I haven't spoken to you for a while, let's chat." Anything to look forward to is a big thing. As I'm writing this, Austin and I are planning a weekend away in Italy. I blocked the days out ages ago. No one gets us that weekend but us.

- Improve your physical situation. Go run until the endorphins kick in. Meditate until you feel centered. Do some yoga until you feel calmly energized. Lift weights until you work up a truly cleansing sweat.

That's my **how-to** on living through suffering. Focus on the positive so firmly that your mind can't see the negative—just for a moment, if that's as much as you can do. Any of these activities, if they work for you, are the right answer.

CONCLUSION

There's a lot of *f#!+* going down.

I don't expect it to decrease in amount, severity, or duration. I expect we'll need to get tougher or smarter about how we deal with turbulent times. Years ago, an early sales training writer, Robert Ringer, devised "The Theory of Sustenance of a Positive Attitude Through the Assumption of a Negative Result."[31] He was a real estate salesman, and wanted to impress on others, both in his field and elsewhere, that we fail most of the time through no fault of our own. In my work, for example, every person successfully placed means other candidates got bad news and many others never even got that far.

Ringer's book, *Winning Through Intimidation*, wasn't written to encourage you to bully people. He updated

---

[31] Robert J. Ringer, *Winning Through Intimidation*. Los Angeles: Stratford Press, 1973.

and retitled the book in 2002 as *To Be or Not to Be Intimidated?* He's acknowledging that failure is part of life—and failure is intimidating—but that each failure brings us closer to success, that the long view is essential to maintaining your positive attitude and motivation.

Ignore or avoid the players who don't subscribe to ethos you believe in. Stand with and be one of the players who embrace and show confidence, lifting others. In so doing, you will, first and foremost, lift yourself. Show up, stand up, speak up.

Then you'll know **Why Brave Woman Win**. You'll be one of them.

APPENDIX — CASE STUDIES

For this study, I asked five women I know and admire—and who I know had to show exemplary bravery at times in their personal and professional lives—to answer some questions about bravery, and for which I am every grateful. I found their answers enlightening and inspiring. I hope you do too, as well. (I've shown their professional role, nationality and location of work to give you an idea of how women everywhere share burdens and solutions through their bravery.)

VALERIE – SENIOR EXECUTIVE IN A GLOBAL ORGANISATION PROTECING WILDLIFE; ZIMBAWEAN, WORKING IN SOUTH AFRICA

- Can you describe a time when you had to choose bravery in your personal or professional life? How did you do it and what did you learn from doing it?

I chose bravery when I had to speak up to some work colleagues on Black Lives Matter in 2021—at the time that George Floyd was murdered in the US. The colleagues did not seem to understand the importance of the protests and the message that the people were demonstrating for. I shared my thoughts in a non-

233

emotional manner that enabled them to see how they were looking at the matter from a place of privilege. I learnt to be brave and to speak up on uncomfortable issues that affect me as a woman of colour and be true to my professionalism. I also learnt that, without the courage to speak up, my colleagues would probably not have had a chance to understand the issue from my perspective and, at least, to empathise with me and other people of colour.

- What does it mean to you to be a role model for others?

To be a role model means that I should consistently demonstrate my values and what I believe in. Also, being a role model, I should be able to be vulnerable and share my feelings about issues without any fear of being judged.

- Can you tell us leaders whom you admire and why? And what does it take for a leader to last?

I admire leaders such as Dr. Iyanla Vanzant and the late Dr. Maya Angelou. These two leaders consistently spread the message of self-awareness and love. They encouraged people to always see the best in others while understanding and leveraging and accepting our differences. They inspire others to be the best that they can in order to give the best in whatever relationship one finds themselves, be it personally or professionally. It takes consistency, empathy, listening and capacity to inspire others for a leader to last.

- What are your personal best habits?

Mindfulness and meditation. I am at my best and feel grounded when I practice these two habits daily.

ANURADHA – SENIOR EXECUTIVE, GLOBAL VACCINE DELIVERY ORGANISATION; INDIAN, WORKING IN GENEVA, SWITZERLAND

- Can you describe a time when you had to choose bravery in your personal or professional life? How did you do it and what did you learn from doing it?

I was appointed as Home Secretary of Chandigarh, a Union Territory in India, in 1995. No woman before me had occupied this high-profile and sensitive position. Chandigarh was the joint capital of two states, Haryana and Punjab. This meant dealing with the highest political and executive echelons of two governments— governments which often pursued different agendas and were often in sharp disagreement.

Militancy in Punjab was at its peak at that time, and its Chief Minister was assassinated by terrorists a few weeks before I took office. There was some skepticism that internal security and law and order could been entrusted to a woman—typically perceived in India as being weaker than men.

I would be untruthful in stating that I was not daunted. However, I was determined to make a success of this challenge and prove that women are as brave as their male counterparts.

What followed in the next four years was unprecedented. As the first female Home Secretary of Chandigarh, I had to ensure a fair and free trial to bring the Chief Minister's assassins to justice. I personally visited the Chandigarh jail where the assassins were held to oversee the very tight security arrangements. Ironically, the assassins managed to escape that high-security prison after I completed my tenure and a male colleague took over.

During this period, I also exposed a large-scale scam which involved siphoning of millions of dollars from publicly-funded construction projects. The racket was run by high-powered interests that included politicians, engineers, investigative agencies and judicial officers. Besides courage, it took a lot of painstaking and thorough work to establish guilt. There were threats, including threats against my life, but I carried on regardless and several senior, powerful officials were successfully charged with corruption.

Chandigarh citizens describe my stint as one of the best and most effective. Led by an honest and courageous female Home Secretary, the city lived and breathed in peace for that time.

This experience taught me several things:

That women would often face skepticism about their abilities, at least initially. It is important that they stay unflappable and confident.

Women must also trust their own instincts and not create self-pressure by imitating their male colleagues.

Women tend to be naturally reflective, fair, and strong. Pursuing their own authentic style can be a great asset.

Family can be an invaluable source of support when women are faced with exceptionally demanding responsibilities. Having a partner and children who buck you up helps you stay on top even when shutters are down.

- What does it mean to you to be a role model for others?

I am filled with pride when I see younger women enthusiastic to fulfill their audacious dreams and drawing some inspiration and strength from my personal journey and stories. Role models are essential to keep hope, optimism and ambition high.

- Can you tell us leaders whom you admire and why? And what does it take for a leader to last?

I am personally inspired by Mother Teresa. To me, she epitomizes absolute courage—not many people in this world can ever touch, let alone serve, the lepers that she dedicated her entire life to helping. To shun all material comforts and luxuries to save and heal the most downtrodden means you have conquered temptation. This is true bravery.

A leader, to last, has to be steadfast—not losing focus on what she sets out to achieve. She has to also lead with character—that is what makes her credible, authentic and inspirational.

- What are your personal best habits?

Selflessness. I am at peace with myself because I do what I love and I love what I do. Nothing else matters.

HANNAH – SENIOR EXECUTIVE IN COMPENSATION & BENEFITS; BRITISH, WORKING IN NEW YORK, NY, USA (AND JILL'S DAUGHTER)

- Can you describe a time when you had to choose bravery in your personal or professional life? How did you do it and what did you learn from doing it?

One particular example is perhaps my greatest bravery challenge. I returned to work after being off for 3 weeks on medical leave and, upon my return, I was pulled into a meeting room and told by my boss that I wasn't "performing" and that I was lucky to get a month's pay in lieu of notice if I signed an agreement to leave the financial firm I worked for in London. This threw me entirely because I had near-perfect reviews from the same person, and had throughout that time what I thought was a good relationship. I had been out on medical leave due to a chronic illness I was born with and had always worked nights and weekends to make up any time off I needed to take for medical leave.

I think the choice to say no to her when she presented me with the separation document—there was no merit to this accusation—and from a woman I thought was a mentor, friend and good boss, was a brave one. The following days of harassment from her also demanded that I be brave in standing up to her. I stood my ground, went to an employment lawyer and learned what she was trying to do was illegal. I was entitled to medical leave, there were no performance issues, but they wanted to 'downsize' me out of the business.

I eventually got a substantial payout for this, but while the money spoke to the injustice of it, I was very happy that I had done what was right, and proved to them they cannot treat others this way.

This process took a few months, and while it was exceptionally stressful, I learnt that you should never let someone bully you into something, especially even when it's someone you formerly trusted. Standing up for yourself doesn't mean you need to be rude, aggressive or dismissive, but you have to stand your ground for what you believe in.

- What does it mean to you to be a role model for others?

To be a role model is to let my actions follow on from my beliefs in what is right, instead of being one who talks but never shows they live their beliefs. My role models lead by example.

- Can you tell us leaders whom you admire and why? And what does it take for a leader to last?

The Prime Minister of New Zealand, Jacinda Ardern, is a great leader actively making a difference in her country. She leads by example. For example, during the pandemic, she postponed her wedding due to

COVID restrictions. Other leaders found ways around the rules, she didn't try. She lived her beliefs.

Mackenzie Scott, most famous as Jeff Bezos' ex-wife, has given over half of her divorce settlement—more than $5 billion—to charity to a variety of causes she supports.

- What are your personal best habits?

Empathy, loyalty, resilience, integrity.

NELA – DIGITAL TRASNFORMATION SPECIALIST; SERBIAN, WORKING IN GREAT BRITAIN

- Can you describe a time when you had to choose bravery in your personal or professional life? How did you do it and what did you learn from doing it?

In 1999, I found myself in war-torn Serbia. During a life-changing 77 days of relentless bombing by NATO, I was presented with an opportunity to escape and start a new life on the other side of the world. Essentially, I was asked if I wanted to step into an unknown with no parachute.

Looking back, that must have been my bravest decision, as I decided to move from Serbia to Australia, leaving all of my family at the age of 17. At the time, I spoke limited English and was facing the final year of high school, with no clear plan of what would happen afterwards.

That decision changed the course of my life. Having successfully navigated this change, I realised that I had enough confidence and resourcefulness to make big life-changing leaps, and that I could thrive in new and challenging situations.

- What does it mean to you to be a role model for others?

Honestly, I'm still struggling with the idea of being a role model for others. But, if I had to choose an example, it has to be taking on the leadership role at work, as the EMEA (Europe, Middle East and Asia) Lead of our Pride community.

Having struggled with my sexuality in private and at work for a number of years in the past, I felt an obligation to put myself forward and be that role model—the successful queer woman that I wish I had been when starting in the corporate world some 17 years ago.

I had to push myself to overcome the "fly under the radar" approach I subscribed to in the past. I started seeking opportunities to put myself under the spot light to share my story and my life. I felt I owed it to my beautiful little family and my soon-to-be-born son.

Soon after I took this role on, I was contacted by a number of LGBTQ+ colleagues and allies that were seeking their tribe and wanted to connect and participate in building our community. I could not be more proud of what this group of motivated people has achieved in less than a year. I feel very humbled by the role I played in it.

- Can you tell us which leaders you admire and why? And what does it take for a leader to last?

Ricardo Semler is the first leader I came across that made me think about leadership. By simply sharing his own leadership philosophy and how he put it into practice in his own company, he redefined the role of a leader for me, as a people-enabler. Apart from running this amazing, human-centric company, Ricardo is also an avid supporter of environmental defense causes in Brazil.

Ursula Burns is another leader that I find very inspiring. She rose through the ranks of Xerox from an intern to the CEO, to became the first black female CEO of a Fortune 500 company. She is also a tireless fighter for equality, and in promoting STEM (Science, Technology, Engineering, Math) education for girls and women.

For a leader to last, they need to be driven by their internal compass, where their north is defined through their own set of values. They can change the sphere of their activity but there is always a common thread, underpinned by their beliefs and the vision of the world. Of course, they need to have high levels of empathy and ability to take their teams on the journey with them, no matter how hazardous it might be.

- What are your personal best habits?

Making and maintaining long-lasting, deep, human connections has always been important to me. As a consequence, I still have friends among my primary school classmates, even though I have lived in five different countries since then.

I make it a habit to reach out to several friends and acquaintances each week. I'm aiming to share the joys and the hard moments of my life with them, even if just via a quick message or call. I find that a small gesture can go a long way.

On a more day-to-day basis, I try to create a sense of routine in the morning—even thought this has been shaken by the arrival of our son, some 5 months ago! I go for a walk before work, during which I get a coffee—a little treat to myself—and I often talk to my mum. This grounds me and feels like a good start to the day.

DEBBIE — FAMILY PSYCHOLOGIST THERAPIST IN PRIVATE PRACTICE; BRITISH, WORKING IN ENGLAND

- Can you describe a time when you had to choose bravery in your personal or professional life? How did you do it and what did you learn from doing it?

Several times, others have told me I'm brave or have been brave to face my challenges: My mother died when I was 11. My first child's birth became a trauma, then the stress of having my second child during my husband's illness. There's never been a choice to be brave at these times, just the choice of carrying on or giving up. Despair and pain are givens (they're part of grief) but this isn't the same as giving up. So, ultimately, for me, this is the life choice for each of us—no matter how complicated a situation might be, there was one basic choice: We can't control the unexpected experiences of birth and death but we can choose how we react to those events, if we want to keep hope within us or give in to the darkness of the event. I decided that, if I lived my life within the constraints of fearing death or endings, it would reduce my hope and life's possibilities.

This decision has cleared a path for me—all that's left to fear are the things that I do have some control over. The bravest steps I've taken have been the times when I've made conscious decisions to go against a narrative or belief about what I am or what my limitations should be. The more I do this the more I realize that it is, ultimately, me that holds me back.

For a long time—throughout school and my early adulthood—I came to believe that part of me wasn't very intelligent. I excelled in creative subjects, had strong friendships, could make people laugh, could tune into ideas about how people might feel, be a trusted confidant to friends, be curious about how people thought or behaved.

I couldn't, however, understand even the most basic mathematical principles. If I managed to learn them, I would immediately forget them. This was astounding, almost to a hilarious degree. While I could laugh it off publicly, I was incredibly frustrated and angry with it privately. A whole section of life that was deemed essential and relatively doable for my peers evaded me.

In primary school, my reports told me that my overall work was of a good standard but that I was incredibly slow and should speed up. For secondary school, I was streamed in a middle set because I excelled in art and English but failed miserably at math. A teacher told me that they put me in the middle because they didn't know where to fit me. After school, I found it near impossible to learn to drive, after taking the test five times in total. To remember or recite directions would cause me to break out in a sweat, if anyone asked details from me. I still slightly dread questions like "Which way did you go?" or "How long will you take?" I struggled to read timetables, grids, spreadsheets, maps, manage money, order numbers. It took me until I was nearly nine to read the time and, even now, analogue is easier because I can see it and divvy it out visually in my mind. I found anything computer-related intensely boring or stressful, as if it was all a language I didn't know. I couldn't easily recite my timetables by the time I was at GCSEs. It was a point of irritation and ridicule for some. This affected my confidence and belief about what I could or couldn't do in my life.

I resigned myself to a belief that I would need to depend upon someone else—or, ultimately, be led by someone else—who knew what "proper life" was really about. The patriarchal narrative around me led me to believe that the skills I did have were not "real intelligence," that the skills I had were best left for the home or general "women's roles," such as motherhood, one day. Certainly, I know these are vital roles, managing a family, raising children well—which is, perhaps, the most challenging of all jobs and the most vital to the fabric of our society and communities. Committed, hardworking parents deserve honor and respect.

Yet, historically, this role has been fed to us as easy, lacking in academic need or real intelligence, not worth paying highly for, but instead, to be given out freely by womankind to benefit the more important roles in life. So, these beliefs around me as a girl and young woman did affect my own beliefs about my potential in life. There were areas where I knew I excelled, so I focused on those, but self-esteem and goals in this other minefield of my life were low. It's these narratives that get built about us that we can take or leave. We don't have to live by them and we certainly don't have to be a prisoner to their limitations. I understand now that if we are brave enough to ask questions, be curious and explore the order of things, we can find the place where we most fit.

Dyscalculia—the inability to understand number concepts—was not really a known condition when I was a child or young adult and, even now, most people may be unaware of it. When someone who had known me for some time kindly mentioned it to me in recent years as a possible reason for some of my struggles, I discovered a new perspective and narrative about myself that finally made sense. I had proof that I wasn't lazy with timekeeping or stupid because I couldn't easily order assignments or decide where things began and ended. Imagine my relief when I could share another narrative—one in which I'm not the patriarchal stereotype of a "ditsy woman" who can't reverse park very well.

So, I journeyed from being the middle child or the creative clown in middle set to qualify as an illustrator and later a family therapist specializing in child and family mental health. I pooled my skills and took brave steps in things where my usual narratives told me I do not excel. I was earning money as a child-minder and cleaner for Jill Bausch when I told her that I wanted to train as a psychotherapist. She helped me navigate the internet—then relatively impossible for me—and wrote me a lovely reference. I got work supporting challenging teenagers in a school and a supervised placement in a family therapy team. Eventually, I qualified with distinction for this along with my practical exam.

I discovered that my difficulties managing 'logical order' were not as important here. For this field, I needed to be able to think outside the box, and in all directions. It demanded that I work with chaos and uncertainty. This was now a skill rather than a disadvantage—family life, feelings, relationships and mental health do not present in an orderly or very logical fashion.

I landed my first therapy job on a wonderful team in a foster agency where I was even given a brand-new company car. Taking that on was brave for me, a big car that I had to drive on the motorway!

Years later, I joined the Child and Adolescent Mental Health Service (CAMHS), working with families, schools, health, and social professionals, offering consultations on children's mental health within that. I was asked to be part of a small pilot project for working with complex family cases and my career took off.

If the old narrative starts raising my anxiety at any point, making me doubt myself, I now know that this is my signal to seriously consider accepting some challenge, to defy my limitations by doing exactly what they tell me I can't. This is my bravery.

- What does it mean to you to be a role model for others?

When we become role models to those we know, we have a responsibility to be true and kind to ourselves, whether we want the responsibility or not. To get to where I am, I've had to believe in and be inspired by other strong women in my life. I'm thrilled that I might be able to do the same for others. There are too many children who are stuck in an ingrained narrative of how girls or boys are expected to behave in order to be liked, accepted, or seen as achieving. I hope that I can help to change that narrative and encourage young people to see themselves as their main USP (Unique Selling Proposition) in life. Warts and all. Particularly the warts!

- Can you tell us leaders whom you admire and why? And what does it take for a leader to last?

I have always admired those who take steps towards liberation or hope even when every narrative or experience around them might be telling them otherwise. Malala Yousafzai (author of *I Am Malala: The Story of the Girl Who Stood Up for Education and was Shot by the Taliban*), Deborah Feldman (*Unorthodox*), Tara Westover (*Educated: A Memoir*), Frank Mc Court (*Angela's Ashes*), Alan Davies (*Just Ignore Him*),

Lemn Sissay (*My Name is Why*) are just some of the superhumans I admire for this.

A true leader and role model needs to be brave enough to ask difficult questions, challenge unhelpful narratives, and provide a safe and compassionate path for others to do the same. Most role models and leaders in my life were never famous. They were simply the strong women who believed in me and showed incredible emotional and mental strength and kindness. Many of these are still close friends, still with me now, while others, like my mother, have passed on.

- What are your personal best habits?

Self-Acceptance, care, and kindness.

Thank you to Valerie, Anuradha, Hannah, Nela and Debbie for your heartfelt stories for sharing your own brave moments.

In closing....

Richard Branson, British entrepreneur and business magnate, from the Sunday Times, UK, 9 July 2022:

"I think being an optimist is a hell of a lot more fun than being a pessimist. As a leader, it's so much better to look for the best in people, to praise people and generally be positive. That brings the best out of people."

Acknowledgements

I wanted to end this book with thoughts about beginnings. Life is always full of new beginnings and without acknowledging those people who have helped me see that, an opportunity would be lost. My endless appreciation and gratitude are warmly given:

To my parents, Josephine, and George Robert, simply for the gift of my being here. And bringing me up with the right values, morals, and confidence we all need.

To my children, Hannah, and Harrison, who have taught me far more about bravery than I have taught them. I am certain there is much more for me to learn from them.

To Austin, who selflessly supported every effort on this project, and who was behind me in every single way possible from the first spark of this idea to the reality of it coming home.

To Pippa, who never gave up in her wise counsel (tempered with lots of laughter), even when others might have.

To all the team at Leaders Press, who unwaveringly helped with so many facets of this book, but especially to Grace, my project manager. The best things in life are often put in front us through serendipity, and Grace is one of them.

To Seamus, who just allowed me to flourish, just as I am, and who always has faith in me because his heart is endless.

To all the women I have coached, mentored, taught, learned from, and the men that support them. Without you I couldn't write a word.

And finally, to all the people who encouraged me to write this book, and those who have now read it. You have given me a gift for which I am extremely grateful. Please now hand your copy of this book to someone else when you are finished, and you will have a piece of sharing inspiration with other brave women.

About Jill Bausch

Jill Bausch is a senior level advisor in Talent Management, Leadership and Social Impact, working across public/ private sectors globally. As head of International Search & Leadership for SRI Executive, she sources high-calibre leaders, creates high-performance teams and advises on organisational structures to achieve maximum social change through creative talent management. She is the former CEO of Futures Group Europe, specialising in behaviour change for social good, is a professor of behaviour change economics, and a specialist in behaviour change and economic empowerment strategies.

She has held international senior talent management roles in North America and Europe and has sourced, managed, trained and coached high-performing executives worldwide in operational and management roles. She is a senior level talent management strategist and facilitator for clients spanning the corporate, public and academic sectors, among them the United Nations network, LVMH Paris, The Green Climate Fund, the Roll Back Malaria Partnership, Apple, The Center for Reproductive Rights, the Organisation for Security & Cooperation in Europe, the World Health Organization, and Gavi, the Vaccine Alliance.

She has built effective teams working across cultures in Asia, Africa, North America and Europe, and is co-founder of VivePoint, coaching and team-building specialists. In addition to her executive search, facilitation and coaching work, she is currently Social Impact Advisor to London Business School, UK; a Business Mentor with the Princes Trust - UK, and former Chair of the Board of Directors, Barefoot College International, working with rural women to improve lives in Asia, Africa and the Pacific Islands. Jill holds an MSc. from the London School of Economics, a B.S. from the University of Cincinnati, is qualified as an Executive Coach through the London Academy of Executive Coaching and is certified in leadership and management assessments including Hogan Personality Assessments and EQi Emotional Intelligence Assessments.

Jill is a dual national of the USA and UK and lives between England and Portugal.

Suggested Reading

1. *Brand You: Turn Your Unique Talents into a Winning Formula* by John Purkiss and David Royston
2. *The 5 Love Languages* by Dr. Gary Chapman (good for leaders to use the principle of understanding what rewards others need and want)
3. *Who: A Method for Hiring* by Geoff Smart and Randy Street (great info on how to communicate effectively when on the job market)
4. *Emotional Intelligence: Why It Can Matter More Than IQ* by Daniel Goleman
5. *TA Today: A New Introduction to Transactional Analysis* by Vann Joines and Ian Stewart (super interesting transactional analysis – regarding how we all have 'scripts' from childhood that we repeat destructively or beneficially as adults)
6. *Wherever You Go, There You Are: Mindfulness Meditation in Everyday Life* by Jon Kabat-Zinn, PhD
7. *The Healing Power of Mindfulness: A New Way of Being* by Jon Kabat-Zinn, PhD
8. *Thinking, Fast and Slow* by Daniel Kahneman (won the nobel prize for literature for this one!)
9. *The EQ Edge: Emotional Intelligence and Your Success* by Steven J. Stein and Howard E. Book

NOTES